100 Quest...
About Panic Disorder

Second Edition

Carol W. Berman, MD

Department of Psychiatry
New York University School of Medicine
New York, NY

JONES AND BARTLETT PUBLISHERS

Sudbury, Massachusetts

BOSTON   TORONTO   LONDON   SINGAPORE

World Headquarters

Jones and Bartlett Publishers
40 Tall Pine Drive
Sudbury, MA 01776
978-443-5000
info@jbpub.com
www.jbpub.com

Jones and Bartlett Publishers
Canada
6339 Ormindale Way
Mississauga, Ontario L5V 1J2
Canada

Jones and Bartlett Publishers
International
Barb House, Barb Mews
London W6 7PA
United Kingdom

Jones and Bartlett's books and products are available through most bookstores and online booksellers. To contact Jones and Bartlett Publishers directly, call 800-832-0034, fax 978-443-8000, or visit our website, www.jbpub.com.

Substantial discounts on bulk quantities of Jones and Bartlett's publications are available to corporations, professional associations, and other qualified organizations. For details and specific discount information, contact the special sales department at Jones and Bartlett via the above contact information or send an email to specialsales@jbpub.com.

The authors, editor, and publisher have made every effort to provide accurate information. However, they are not responsible for errors, omissions, or for any outcomes related to the use of the contents of this book and take no responsibility for the use of the products and procedures described. Treatments and side effects described in this book may not be applicable to all people; likewise, some people may require a dose or experience a side effect that is not described herein. Drugs and medical devices are discussed that may have limited availability controlled by the Food and Drug Administration (FDA) for use only in a research study or clinical trial. Research, clinical practice, and government regulations often change the accepted standard in this field. When consideration is being given to use of any drug in the clinical setting, the healthcare provider or reader is responsible for determining FDA status of the drug, reading the package insert, and reviewing prescribing information for the most up-to-date recommendations on dose, precautions, and contraindications, and determining the appropriate usage for the product. This is especially important in the case of drugs that are new or seldom used.

Production Credits

Senior Acquisition Editor: Alison Hankey
Editorial Assistant: Sara Cameron
Production Director: Amy Rose
Production Editor: Dan Stone
Marketing Manager: Ilana Goddess

V.P. of Manufacturing and Inventory Control:
    Therese Connell
Composition: Spoke & Wheel/Jason Miranda
Printing and Binding: Malloy, Inc.

Cover Credits

Cover Design: Carolyn Downer
Cover Image: © Carol W. Berman, MD
Cover Printing: Malloy, Inc.

Library of Congress Cataloging-in-Publication Data

Berman, Carol W.
    100 questions & answers about panic disorder / Carol W. Berman. — 2nd ed.
       p. cm.
    Includes bibliographical references and index.
    ISBN-13: 978-0-7637-7523-0
    1. Panic disorders—Popular works. 2. Panic disorders—Miscellanea. I. Title. II. Title: One hundred questions and answers about panic disorder.
    RC535.B475 2009
    616.85'223—dc22
                                     2009007077
6048

Printed in the United States of America
13 12 11 10 09   10 9 8 7 6 5 4 3 2 1

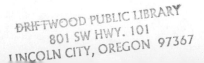

Almost everyone feels anxious at times. Anxiety is a common experience, particularly as a response to life stresses. However, severe and uncontrollable anxiety can become a disabling condition. Community studies indicate that 19% of men and 31% of women will develop some type of anxiety disorder during their lifetime.[1] According to recent census estimates, more than 20 million American adults experienced an anxiety disorder at some point in their lives.

A panic attack involves such a high level of anxiety that the person affected feels as if he or she can't breathe, is having a heart attack, going insane, or losing control. Other typical symptoms include tingling sensations, ringing in the ears, trembling, a feeling of choking, chest pain, sweating, and heart pounding. Many individuals even experience panic that awakens them from sleep, so-called "nocturnal panic attacks." In any given year, 30% to 40% of the general population will have a panic attack. Fortunately, most of these individuals will not go on to develop panic disorder, which has a lifetime prevalence of approximately 3.5%.[1] Of those who do develop panic disorder, many also experience agoraphobia, which is fear of places or situations where a panic attack may occur or from which escape might be difficult in the event of a panic attack. For example, people with agoraphobia often avoid being out alone, going to supermarkets, traveling in trains or airplanes, crossing bridges, climbing to heights, going through tunnels, crossing open fields, and riding in elevators. Agoraphobia takes a toll not only on those afflicted, but on their friends and loved ones, who often are called upon to accompany them on everyday tasks and errands.

100 Questions & Answers About Panic Disorder, Second Edition by Carol W. Berman, MD, fills an important need for those affected by panic attacks—as well as for their friends, families, employers, coworkers, and anyone else who simply wants to better understand this common and sometimes disabling condition. Written for a lay audience in a clear and succinct style, the

---

[1] Kessler R, McGonagle K, Zhao S, et al. Lifetime and 12-month prevalence of DSM-III-R psychiatric disorders in the United States. Results from the National Comorbidity Survey. *Arch Gen Psychiatry* 1994; 51:8–19.

book addresses the most common—and even some less common but very compelling—questions surrounding this condition. Free of technical jargon (unless accompanied by explanation), it covers all aspects of panic attacks including diagnosis, etiology, course of illness, coping strategies, and treatment. It answers those questions that you may have been too timid to ask of your doctor, or forgot to ask, or simply ran out of time to ask! At the end of the book are useful references to organizations and web sites for more information, as well as prevention strategies, lists of medications, and types of talk therapies used in the treatment of this condition.

An experienced psychopharmacologist, Dr. Berman is also a gifted author and playwright, which makes her well-suited to take on the task of not only elucidating all dimensions of panic attacks, but of making her book an interesting read as well. In this concise volume, she demonstrates a clinician's knack for ferreting out those questions most relevant to patients and their families, a scientist's understanding of the pathophysiology and treatment of this disease, and a writer's gift to synthesize and transmit all of this highly complex information in an informative, entertaining, and easy-to-understand manner.

For anyone who may be suffering from panic attacks (or their loved ones), the good news is that there are very effective treatments available for this condition, making it one of the "success stories" of modern medicine. This book is a welcome addition to the field that is sure to be valued by clinicians and patients for years to come.

David L. Ginsberg, MD
Clinical Associate Professor
Department of Psychiatry
New York University School of Medicine
New York, New York

You are sitting at your work desk minding your own business when out of the blue, a dreadful feeling rises out of your chest into your throat. Your heart is racing. You can't breathe. You sweat, shake, and get dizzy. As you clutch your chair to steady yourself, you think, "What's going on? Am I going crazy?"

The answer is you are having a panic attack. You're not alone. About 2% of the American population has them also, which is 1 out of every 50 people. The good news is that many medications and therapies are available to help you. This book, *100 Questions & Answers About Panic Disorder, Second Edition,* was written to answer many of your questions.

I am a physician who specializes in psychiatry. I treat many patients who suffer from panic disorder. Each new patient with panic attacks has a 90% chance to be panic attack-free in a month or sooner with the right treatment. Not all people suffering from mental disorders are as fortunate as panic attack patients, who usually have such a good prognosis. In the cases of schizophrenia or obsessive-compulsive disorder, for example, there is a much lower rate of successful treatment.

In panic disorder, the worst problem is the fear of panic attacks themselves. This fear often causes agoraphobia, a condition where the patient is too frightened to go outside. As you read this book, you will gain an understanding of what panic attacks are, how the brain sends a false alarm to the body, how to combat panic attacks, how to keep them away, and what follow-up treatment is necessary. Knowing about the characteristics of panic attacks will help you reduce the fear.

Marvin, my patient and commentator, was severely disturbed by his panic attacks. At first he couldn't imagine what was happening to him. Once he was armed with information about his condition, however, he was able to accept treatment, medication, and psychotherapy. Today he is free from panic attacks and is enjoying his life to the fullest.

Carol W. Berman, MD

PART ONE

The Basics

What is a panic attack?

Why do I feel like running away when
I have a panic attack?

I've always been an anxious person. How do these
panic attacks differ from my usual anxiety?

More . . .

1. What is a panic attack?

A panic attack is a discrete episode of anxiety. It may be accompanied by a racing or pounding heart, sweating, trembling or shaking, sensations of shortness of breath, choking feelings, chest pain or discomfort, nausea, stomach ache, dizziness or faintness, derealization, depersonalization, a feeling of losing control or of going crazy, overwhelming fear of death, tingling, chills or "hot flushes." To be classified as an "official" panic attack, see **Table 1** from the *Diagnostic and Statistical Manual of Mental Disorders, Fourth Edition (DSM-IV)*. The *DSM-IV* is a reference book containing the classification of mental disorders used by most psychiatrists, psychologists, social workers, and other mental health professionals. According to the *DSM-IV*, a panic attack must have at least four of the symptoms listed in Table 1, and they must develop abruptly and reach a peak in ten minutes or less. Few people will get all of these symptoms, although some do. Most patients will feel about five symptoms. A panic attack should not be confused with an **anxiety attack**, which doesn't have to be a discrete episode of anxiety with the above symptoms, but can be excessive worry with muscle tension, shakiness, shortness of breath, dizziness, and so forth. Often a panic attack just consists of a pounding heart, dizziness, a feeling of losing control, and hot flushes. If you don't know that this is a panic attack, it can be even more frightening. Patients are even taken to the emergency room (ER) because they believe they are having a heart attack or some other serious medical condition. Once you know it's a panic attack, you can practice breathing exercises or adjust medications to modify the attack. If you have an attack that has fewer than four symptoms, you might be having a limited-symptom attack, but it is still a type of panic attack. For you to be diagnosed with panic disorder,

Diagnostic and Statistical Manual of Mental Disorders, Fourth Edition (DSM-IV)

Reference textbook of classifications used by mental health professionals to diagnose people with mental disorders.

Anxiety attack

An episode of fear that is not as defined as a panic attack and doesn't have to occur out of the blue as most panic attacks do.

Table 1 Characteristics of a Panic Attack

Definition: A discrete period of intense fear or discomfort, in which four (or more) of the following symptoms develop abruptly and reach a peak within 10 minutes:

1. Palpitations, pounding heart, or accelerated heart rate
2. Sweating
3. Trembling or shaking
4. Sensations of shortness of breath or smothering
5. Feeling of choking
6. Chest pain or discomfort
7. Nausea or abdominal distress
8. Feeling dizzy, unsteady, lightheaded, or faint
9. Derealization (feelings of unreality) or depersonalization (being detached from oneself)
10. Fear of losing control or going crazy
11. Fear of dying
12. Paresthesias (numbness or tingling sensations)
13. Chills or hot flushes

Reprinted with permission from *Diagnostic and Statistical Manual of Mental Disorders, Text Revision, Fourth Edition*, (Copyright 2000). American Psychiatric Association.

THE BASICS

you need to have recurrent, unexpected panic attacks, and then at least one month of concern about having panic attacks with all the implications and consequences. If you aren't worried about panic attacks, you don't have panic disorder. Panic attack patients are always concerned about the possibility of another attack even when they've been panic attack-free for some time.

If you aren't worried about panic attacks, you don't have panic disorder.

Marvin's comments:

When I had panic attacks, they only consisted of a pounding heart, dizziness, a stomachache, and a horrible fear of dying. As Dr. Berman says, you just need four of the symptoms she has listed in Table 1. My four symptoms were enough for me. If I would have had anything more, I wouldn't have been able to stand it. The first time I had a panic attack I was driving in my car over a bridge. I pulled over to the side of the road and clutched my chest for many minutes before I could even look up. I thought my time had come to die, even though I was only 38. I wanted to go to the ER, but I knew that was a hassle because my girlfriend, a nurse, told me that you had to wait hours to see a doctor. I didn't think I could handle waiting in my condition, so I sweated it out by myself. The second time I had a panic attack (a few days later), I made an appointment with my G.P. I couldn't believe it when he told me that I was O.K. I certainly didn't feel O.K. until Dr. Berman made the diagnosis of panic attacks and started me on Celexa®, which helped in two weeks. The best thing was to know that those horrible feelings had a name and a treatment.

2. Why do I feel like running away when I have a panic attack?

Epinephrine

A chemical hormone released in the body after a stress stimulus, also called adrenaline, it is a "fight or flight" chemical that makes a person able to flee or fight an enemy or danger.

Adrenaline

A hormone released into the body that stimulates the physiological response of fear and anxiety (also, called epinephrine).

When you have a panic attack, **epinephrine** is released by the body and floods your system. Otherwise known as **adrenaline**, epinephrine is a "fight or flight" chemical that makes a person able to flee or fight an enemy or danger, a very useful characteristic for human survival. Whenever excessive adrenaline is in your body, the effect is to supply more sugar to muscle tissue, make you breathe harder, and prepare you for action, so of course you are ready to run. However, there is usually no immediate danger to you, since a panic attack is a false alarm (see Question 6). Instead of running away, you should try to sit down, breathe deeply, and use cognitive behavioral therapy (CBT) techniques (described in Question 41). Giving in to the impulse to run away is usually a mistake.

A patient of mine was riding on a city bus when she had a severe panic attack. At the time she didn't know what was wrong. She followed her instinct to flee and wound up breaking her ankle. Needless to say, the pain, suffering, and loss of time and income could have been avoided if she would have resisted her strong impulse to run. Now that she realizes she has panic disorder, she is able to control herself and not run. In addition, she has very few panic attacks because her medications are effective.

Other patients have fled boats, subway cars, theaters, and other places. The feelings usually involve the belief that the person will be trapped in some small space, and experience the horrible fear of a panic attack. Running away doesn't stop the actual symptoms of the panic attack, but people distract themselves by running. However, by the time they have "escaped," the panic attack has ended because it would have been over anyway in a few minutes.

3. I've always been an anxious person. How do these panic attacks differ from my usual anxiety?

It is important to remember that a panic attack is a discrete, contained episode of anxiety, unlike generalized anxiety, which can last anywhere from an hour to a lifetime.

Anxiety can cause a pounding heart and other bodily sensations, like sweating, tension, and increased pulse. It is the fear of danger and the feeling of an inability to cope with that anticipated danger. Most people have anxiety. Anxiety can protect people from actual problems, but in many cases it causes individuals to lead a constricted, uncomfortable life. Many journalists have written articles about our current era, calling it the "age of anxiety." Anxiety disorders are the most common disorders seen in psychiatry, and anxiety is a component of all psychiatric illnesses, especially panic disorder. The number of illnesses with anxiety as the basis is startling. These include obsessive-compulsive disorder, social phobia, posttraumatic stress disorder, generalized anxiety disorder, agoraphobia, and substance-induced anxiety disorder, among others. Our treatments for anxiety need to expand. Presently, the medications and various psychotherapies in use are not always adequate. The good news is that the medications we have to treat panic disorder are very effective, more so than for most other anxiety problems. Panic disorder itself is easier to resolve than generalized anxiety disorder, obsessive-compulsive disorder, and social phobia. Once a person is given an anti-anxiety medication, like Xanax®, and a **selective serotonin reuptake inhibitor (SSRI)**, like Zoloft®, the panic attacks can be controlled in a few days. In generalized anxiety disorder, a patient may take these two medicines plus have psychotherapy for years and still suffer from the condition. In terms of treatment, it's almost better to have panic disorder than anything else, although it may feel much worse temporarily.

Marvin's comments:

I've always been an anxious person too. Since I was a kid, I had sweaty palms and a knot in my stomach, but these panic attacks were way beyond any anxiety you can imagine. On a scale of one to ten, I'd been living with a "two or three" anxiety level and a panic attack was a "ten" or more. Panic attacks didn't feel related to ordinary anxiety. They were unique, over-the-top. I can relate to the patient who ran off the bus and broke her ankle. During a panic attack I've run out of places too. It's easy to want to believe that the problem is outside of yourself and try to run from it. Therapy helped me to get in touch with my real feelings and ease my anxieties.

Selective serotonin reuptake inhibitors (SSRIs)

A type of antidepressant that doesn't allow serotonin to be taken up again by neuroreceptors, thereby causing more serotonin to be present to the neurons, which decreases panic attacks; includes drugs such as Prozac®, Zoloft®, Paxil®, Celexa®, Luvox®, and Lexapro®.

4. What is derealization?

Derealization is a feeling of unreality or altered reality, to which panic attack patients are subject. Sometimes people feel they are in a dream or in another dimension. They feel that what is happening is not real. Schizophrenics or those with drug reactions can suffer from derealization as well. A panic attack patient is especially frightened of derealization because she is trying to hold on to reality as strongly as possible and it seems to be escaping from her.

One of my patients would view other people on the subway as automatons whenever she had a panic attack. These episodes of derealization were extremely upsetting, because she never wanted to feel that isolated from others and to consider other people as just a bunch of robots going through mechanical maneuvers. Once her medications were in order, these episodes of derealization became infrequent.

Schizophrenics can easily see other people as robots or machines, but they would be less troubled than panic attack patients by the phenomenon. Drug-induced derealization episodes would also be better tolerated because patients would realize that they were transitory. In fact, some people take drugs, for example, marijuana or LSD, to voluntarily experience removal from reality. To them, reality is too harsh and they would rather be in a dream world.

Most panic attack patients are extremely fearful of losing contact with reality, so they don't drink or take drugs in the first place. Thus, when they experience derealization, they are more upset than anyone else. Fear itself can cause the body to secrete chemicals that make a

Derealization
A feeling of unreality or altered reality.

THE BASICS

Fear itself can cause the body to secrete chemicals that make a person feel spaced out or unreal.

person feel spaced out or unreal. During therapy, psychiatrists or psychologists can teach patients how to ground themselves through breathing and other exercises so they won't experience derealization.

5. What is depersonalization?

Depersonalization

State of not feeling like oneself or feeling alienated from one's own behavior.

Depersonalization is the state of not feeling like oneself or feeling alienated from one's own behavior. Panic attack patients say that they feel they are watching themselves from outside of themselves.

I had a panic attack patient who felt constantly depersonalized. He never believed that he was inside of his own perspective, but instead felt he was always "outside of himself." He always knew reality from unreality, but he couldn't shake this strange feeling. He was very distressed by this state of mind and spent a lot of his time obsessing about it. His hands and feet felt bigger than normal, and he believed he was dragging himself around. To look at him, one did not notice any abnormalities. He was not a schizophrenic nor did he have a dissociative disorder. I sent him to a neurologist, who ruled out migraine headaches, brain tumors, and such. An internist assured me that the patient didn't have hypoglycemia (low blood sugar) or hypothyroidism (low thyroid functioning). Finally, we concluded that he had panic disorder with depersonalization. He refused any medications and stopped psychotherapy so he couldn't be treated anymore.

Most people do not have such extreme cases of depersonalization. Panic attack patients usually go in and out of periods of depersonalization that is consistently associated with panic attacks themselves. If you experience depersonalization, the best way to treat it is to assure yourself that everything is O.K. and you will be yourself soon. Fear can drive you into feeling spaced out and not in your body. If you sit down and hold on to a solid object like a wooden table or something similar while you take deep breaths, you will soon feel like yourself. Hardly anyone continues to feel depersonalized for very long. The patient just described is a rare exception.

6. What causes panic attacks?

One theory has it that panic attacks are caused by a falsely activated alarm system in the brain. This area is called the **locus ceruleus** because the neurons there are blue in color (**Figure 1**). The major concentration of **adrenergic** (adrenaline-like) neurons is located in the locus ceruleus. The axons (which are parts of the nerve cell that conduct the nervous impulses away from the

Locus ceruleus

Part of the brain that contains the major concentration of adrenergic (adrenaline-like) neurons.

Adrenergic

Having to do with nerve pathways in which transmission is with epinephrine (adrenaline) or norepinephrine.

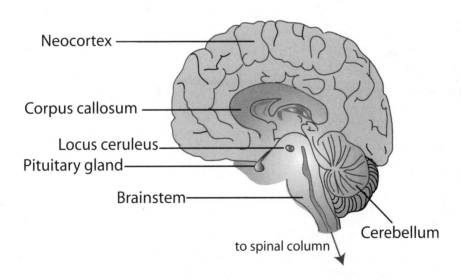

Neocortex

Corpus callosum

Locus ceruleus
Pituitary gland

Brainstem

to spinal column

Cerebellum

Figure 1 Basic structures of the human brain.

Thalamus

A part of the brain that has to do with pain and some emotions.

Hypothalamus

An area of the brain below the thalamus involved in the control of the nervous system and certain hormones.

Panic attacks are caused by chemical imbalances in the nervous system and not by a patient's imagination

Hippocampus

A region of the temporal lobe of the brain that controls learning and memory.

Limbic system

A group of brain parts located below the cortex that is concerned with emotion and motivation.

Neuroreceptors

A structural protein molecule on the nerve cell that binds to a specific factor, such as a neurotransmitter.

cell body) of these nerve cells are connected into the cerebral cortex, the limbic system, the **thalamus**, and the **hypothalamus**. A person has noradrenergic overload when the false alarm goes off. Panic attack patients are then flooded with adrenaline (epinephrine), which makes them feel frightened and triggers a "fight or flight" response when nothing bad is actually happening in the environment. Early human beings developed these biological systems when they needed to either defend themselves from an enemy or escape immediately from dangerous situations. Like any alarm system, it's easy for it to go astray. The malfunction of the system is thought to be hereditary. Lately, data are also showing that panic attacks are caused by abnormalities in certain GABA (γ-aminobutyric acid) or serotonin systems of the brain. Clearly, panic attacks are caused by chemical imbalances in the nervous system and not by a patient's imagination, as many people might claim. The exact cause or causes of panic attacks remain unknown. The **hippocampus** is an elongated structure in the floor of the ventricle of the brain that is an important part of the limbic system. The **limbic system** is a group of brain parts located below the cortex that is concerned with emotion and motivation. It is not clear if this area of the brain is involved in panic disorder. More research is needed to understand these areas. At any rate, we would not say that you are "brain damaged" if you have panic attacks, but you can say that your alarm system is faulty. When a person takes antidepressants, we believe that these medicines get into the locus ceruleus part of the brain and down-regulate **neuroreceptors**. Down-regulation of receptors may be a healing process of the faulty alarm system. In about 50% of cases, treatment of panic attacks with antidepressants for one year will lead to a panic attack-free life afterwards.

Marvin's comments:

It's good to know that panic attacks have a physical cause and are not just in your imagination. Many times I felt bad because I thought I was imagining my panicky feelings. I tried to will them away—to tell myself to snap out of it, but I couldn't. It made me feel terrible about myself. I like this analogy Dr. Berman uses about a house with a faulty alarm system. That's easy to visualize. I don't blame myself as much if I believe I just have a bad alarm system. Maybe someday they'll fix this part of the brain where the problem originates. Also, I don't have to criticize my parents for bringing me up the wrong way if I consider the problem a physical or chemical imbalance. I'm fond of my parents and would rather credit them for bringing me up correctly.

7. Can I die from panic attacks?

A person cannot die from panic attacks, although often people having panic attacks feel as though they might die. Many times patients are brought to the emergency room because they fear they're having a heart attack. When an **electrocardiogram (EKG)** and blood tests are taken, it's found that no physical damage has been done, even though the person may have had sensations of tingling in the arms or chest pain similar to a heart attack. The false alarm that goes off in the brain makes a person believe he is dying. Fear is the main element with which a panic attack patient must deal. Once the diagnosis has been made and treatment started, anxiety decreases and the chance that someone will fear that he is dying from a panic attack will be minimal. There is nothing particularly dangerous about having a panic attack. It is not harmful for the brain and body to be flooded by

Electrocardiogram (EKG)

An electrical record of the heart which shows the heart's integrated action currents; useful test to rule out cardiovascular problems or disease.

There is nothing particularly dangerous about having a panic attack.

adrenaline. It is a common condition to which a person can accommodate himself or herself. Of course, panic attack patients are terrified to be in this state, but once they learn that they won't have any physical problems as a consequence, they usually feel better and adapt to the condition. Fear of dying and losing control are the primary fears in panic disorder. The panic attack patient is overly controlled as a consequence. Treatment consists of "loosening up" the panic attack patient through deep breathing, relaxation techniques, and getting the person in touch with his emotional state. The excessive control that the panic attack patient exercises over himself does not allow him to feel his emotions fully.

8. Why does my heart race or pound during a panic attack?

During a panic attack, a shot of adrenaline courses through the body. The adrenaline (epinephrine) causes nerves to stimulate the heart. The heart pumps faster so that the endangered person has enough strength to "fight or flee." The only problem is that there is no danger. Most patients have increased anxiety when they experience **palpitations**, which is an awareness of the beating of the heart brought about by change in the heart's rhythm or rate. Palpitations do not indicate any particular group of cardiac disorders. When cardiologists hear their patients describing "pounding," "racing," "fluttering," or "flopping" hearts, they think about psychiatric causes. Patients with anxiety show a greater awareness of changes in their heart's rhythm and rate. People with organic heart disease tend to grow accustomed to these abnormalities, and they often are less aware than anxious people of their hearts. The chances are that if you aware

Palpitations

Awareness of the beating of the heart brought about by change in the heart's rhythm or rate.

of your heart and worried about it, you are experiencing psychiatric problems and not cardiac ones. The idea is to not obsess about your heart if you feel it racing. Just relax and understand that it's a part of normal functioning. When EKGs and other tests are done, you will be able to see that nothing is wrong with your heart, and that it is only panic.

9. Can I faint from a panic attack?

It's unlikely that you will faint during a panic attack, but people often feel dizzy. One should try to breathe normally and not hyperventilate, a process that causes dizziness and faintness in the first place. I've only heard of a few patients fainting while having a panic attack. Syncope or fainting may be what is called a **vasovagal response**, which is an action of the vagus nerve on the blood vessels. This is the most common faint experienced by normal people. It can happen during emotional stress, like a panic attack, especially in a warm, crowded room. Physiologically, there is a big drop in blood pressure. Cardiac output is normal, but it fails to increase blood pressure in response to the drop as it usually would. The vagus nerve to the heart causes heart slowing (**bradycardia**), and then an increase in heart rate (**tachycardia**), further lowering of blood pressure, and a reduction in blood to the brain. The person faints. Fainting is not dangerous unless one hits one's head on something. Usually people don't faint during a panic attack, but they worry that they will faint. Drinking a glass of water may often abort a faint because it takes a person's mind off fear.

Vasovagal response

An action of the vagus nerve on the blood vessels. This is the most common faint experienced by normal people. It can happen during emotional stress.

Bradycardia

A slow heartbeat, under 60 beats/minute.

Tachycardia

A fast heartbeat.

10. Why do I blush when I have a panic attack?

Blushing, a sudden and brief redness of the face and neck due to emotion, commonly happens when panic attacks are related to social or performance anxiety. Many people have this condition without having panic attacks. They become excessively frightened of giving speeches or performing in front of an audience (i.e., "stage fright"), or sometimes it will just happen with everyday social interactions. If they are blushing, it is even more embarrassing because people can actually see their shame or other emotion. A blush is caused by **vasodilation**, or widening of the blood vessels, at the skin surface. Perhaps it's also due to an increase in adrenaline.

Vasodilation

A widening of the blood vessels at the skin surface, causing a flush or blush; may be due to an increase in adrenaline.

For those with panic attacks, blushing may be one of the most embarrassing symptoms because you feel that people are able to detect that you are having a panic attack. I tell my patients that most people in an audience are not scrutinizing the speaker, as panic attack patients believe. Often audience members do not notice small details like a blush coming over your skin. The main idea is to concentrate on your speech and disregard various bodily sensations, like blushing, palpitations, and so forth. Panic attack patients have been shown to obsess about various sensations that most people ignore. Excessive focusing on these elements causes more anxiety and can actually induce a panic attack. Relaxation techniques and medications can help with these problems. When audience members are interviewed about whether or not a speaker blushed or trembled, most of them cannot remember. In other words, people are not aware of small details indicating the nervousness of the speaker. The speaker is hyperaware of his own anxiety, especially if he or she suffers from panic disorder. It's helpful to know that those observing you are unaware of these things.

11. I found that if I'm up on a high mountain or in an area of low oxygen, I could have a panic attack. Why?

Panic attacks have been associated with low oxygen in the body (O_2) or high carbon dioxide (CO_2). The reason is not clear, but it may be that the faulty alarm system in the brain that causes panic attacks is fired by low O_2, high CO_2. One of the old techniques for aborting a panic attack, before we had such effective medications, was to have the person breathe into a paper bag. In this way the panic attack patient was exposed to decreased **hyperventilation** and often the panic attack would stop. Breathing into a paper bag would drive the respiratory system toward higher oxygen levels, too. However, the respiratory system would not be able to compensate and increase O_2 and lower CO_2 very much if the person was located in a high altitude environment like the Rocky Mountains. So breathing into a paper bag there would not be helpful. Perhaps this technique would also distract the patient from his extreme fear until the panic attack would be over. Panic attack sufferers are notorious hyperventilators, which could be caused by higher adrenaline levels in the blood. Learning proper breathing and behavioral therapy can help. If you find yourself hyperventilating and feeling panicky, lie down, put your hands on your stomach and force yourself to breathe very slowly. As you inhale deeply, experience your hands raising up on your belly. When you exhale, press your stomach in and try to breathe out as much air as you can. In this manner you can stop a rapid breathing pattern and derail a panic attack.

Hyperventilation
Short, shallow, rapid breaths.

12. I was molested as a child. Is this the reason I have panic attacks now as an adult?

Any kind of early trauma can contribute to the development of panic disorder.

Any kind of early trauma can contribute to the development of panic disorder, because we believe it causes excessive stimulation of brain centers that control epinephrine and serotonin production and actually changes brain chemistry. Patients who have a history of early trauma often go see their doctors with panic attacks. After we gain control of the panic attacks, we can begin to work on the original problems such as molestation or any other kind of early trauma. Psychotherapy with panic attack patients while they are in the throes of the attacks is too difficult. We are fortunate to have many medications and other techniques to control, and in many cases eliminate, panic attacks completely. It is believed that the SSRIs and other antidepressants that we use for treatment of panic attacks are capable of changing the noradrenergic and serotonergic systems of the brain that were stressed by the trauma. Sometimes these changes are permanent and helpful to panic attack patients. There are no claims that we can restore the brain to a pre-trauma condition, but that is not necessary. In some cases, psychotherapy and behavioral treatment can alter brain chemistry positively, too. Having to hide early trauma, like molestation, can keep a person in a state of **vigilance** and anxiety. This constant stressful state is a strain on the nervous system, leading to panic and other disorders. Psychotherapy releases the patient from this emotional prison, allowing resolution. Many panic attack patients have been living in constant dread. They are relieved to finally deal with these issues.

Vigilance

A constant stressful state that strains the nervous system, leading to anxiety, panic, and other disorders.

13. What is agoraphobia?

Agoraphobia is anxiety about going or being outside and/or avoidance of certain places or situations where it might be difficult or embarrassing to escape. Agoraphobics are afraid of being outside their homes alone, being in a crowd, standing in a line, being on a bridge, or of traveling in a bus, train, or car.

Often panic attacks occur and then lead a person to become agoraphobic. Outside places are associated with panic attacks, and patients become **phobic** of these places. Some individuals are able to expose themselves to these places, but they feel terrible dread while they are there and can't wait to escape. Many patients are able to tolerate being in a feared place if accompanied by a companion. Many panic attack patients feel they can't handle the outside world by themselves because they might faint, "go crazy," or otherwise be incapacitated. They believe the companion will rescue them if something happens.

However, when patients avoid situations, they impair their ability to travel, work, and carry out homemaking responsibilities. Some people wind up completely housebound. Every environment, including hallways, elevators, and staircases, becomes a problem. In that case, behavioral psychologists may have to go into a person's home and **de-condition** the person to help him or her out of the house.

I had one patient who bravely fought against agoraphobia for ten years. Finally, after a severe flu episode, she became trapped in her apartment and could no longer

Agoraphobia

Anxiety about going or being outside and/or avoidance of certain places or situations where it might be difficult or embarrassing to escape.

Phobia

An objectively unfounded, morbid dread or fear that arouses a state of panic; used in combination with the object that inspires the fear.

De-condition

To change or eliminate a conditioned (learned) response.

go to the office to work. When she had to go to the doctor for her heart condition, her son held her around the waist, led her down the stairs, and took her in by the hand to the doctor who was only four blocks from her apartment. Every step was excruciating, and she tried to keep her eyes closed the whole time she was outdoors.

Marvin's comments:

I have agoraphobia too. On the weekends I can stay in all day on Saturday and Sunday. Not going outside makes me feel safe and comfortable, but then I feel distressed that I'm not going to the gym or doing necessary chores. Dr. Berman always encouraged me to force myself to go outside, even if I felt I couldn't. That was the best advice. These days I don't have panic attacks, so it's much easier to fight agoraphobia, but I also counteract it by planning my schedule on the weekend. Saturday I start with a basketball game, followed by lunch with teammates. Afterwards, I do my food shopping, reserve time for relaxing in the backyard, and finally try to get out to a movie. Sunday I've been taking a class on organizing my finances. Having a schedule helps you get out.

14. Should I avoid having children if I have panic attacks?

First-degree biological relatives of panic disorder patients (like children) have a four to seven times greater chance of developing it than the rest of the population. However, as many as 50% to 75% of individuals with panic attacks do not have an affected first-degree biological relative. Whether or not to have children is always a personal choice. Since the scientific community has not definitely identified the **gene** or genes responsible for panic attacks, we cannot see if a fetus has those genes in the same manner as we can look for a gene like, for example,

Gene

A DNA sequence that codes for a protein, genes are the biological basis of hereditiy.

Tay Sachs disease. Some individuals with Tay Sachs or other dangerous medical disorders forego having children because they don't want to pass these genes on to the next generation. However, in the future, gene technology might advance to the point where those genes could be altered and eliminate the diseases before the baby is born. We are already doing such operations with cystic fibrosis babies. Surgeons are able to fix their genes and help the babies to live longer. Panic disorder is not as disabling as Tay Sachs or cystic fibrosis. Also, there is no evidence that everyone born with the gene or genes will develop the condition of panic disorder. However, the issue is really your choice to have or not to have children after getting all of the facts. Most panic attack patients can look back at the family tree and identify a mother, grandmother, or aunt who had or has panic disorder. People often remember female relatives with it, since females seem to be affected more than males. We are looking forward to the time when we'll be able to eliminate panic attacks medically and genetically.

There is no evidence that everyone born with the gene or genes will develop the condition of panic disorder.

PART TWO

Risks and Causes

Why do I get panic attacks after I drink coffee?

If I don't get enough sleep (less than 6 hours),
I find I can have a panic attack. Why?

Should I avoid alcohol if I have panic disorder?

More . . .

15. Why do I get panic attacks after I drink coffee?

Coffee and other stimulants activate central nervous system pathways that cause panic attacks. Once patients have been medicated, they may be able to return to coffee drinking, but at the beginning of diagnosis and treatment it is better to stay away from all caffeinated drinks, including colas and teas. Herbal teas are caffeine-free, but sometimes they contain other chemicals that might trigger panic attacks, such as ephedra. One should always read labels very carefully to see what is being consumed. If you have been panic attack-free for some time and then re-develop them after eating or drinking something, you should bring that product to your psychiatrist, who can help you figure out what the offending substance might be. Ma Huang, for example, is a Chinese herb that contains ephedra, which is known to cause nervous excitability. Avoid that. Yerba Maté is a stimulant from South America that people in that country use instead of or in addition to coffee. Panic attack patients should be careful not to ingest any of these herbs, and if they do, they should realize they may get a panic attack.

At the beginning of diagnosis and treatment, it is better to stay away from all caffeinated drinks.

Marvin's comments:

I have no problem drinking coffee. In fact, if I don't drink coffee, I feel panicky or withdrawal effects. I understand that a lot of people have different anxiety reactions to coffee, tea, or chocolate. I'm pretty much normal when it comes to foods, but I have funny reactions to medicines. One time I tried Benadryl® to help me sleep. The doctor told me it was harmless, but it caused me to have a panic attack. From then on I stayed away from it. Each person has to be aware of his own reactions and respect them.

16. If I don't get enough sleep (less than 6 hours), I find I can have a panic attack. Why?

Lack of sleep may stimulate certain hormones or other chemicals in the body to cause panic attacks. The best plan is to try to eat and sleep well and have as regular a lifestyle as possible when dealing with panic disorder. One patient, a student, stayed up studying until 4 AM each night. She would wake up at 8:30 AM, skip breakfast, and dash out to classes. When her panic attacks started, she became frightened of going to sleep and often would stay up all night, dreading even getting into bed to try to sleep. Her panic attacks worsened as she built up a sleep deficit. Finally, she sought treatment. She was given a sleep-inducing antidepressant, Zoloft®, and advised to go to bed by midnight at the latest and awaken at eight. She followed this advice, obtaining good results. Even before her antidepressant worked (three weeks), she felt rested and had a decrease in the number of panic attacks she experienced. She knew she had to eat regularly while taking Zoloft®, so she instituted a regular breakfast, lunch, and dinner schedule. In two months she thought that she was "cured" since she didn't experience any panic attacks and returned to her old schedule of not eating or sleeping regularly. Her panic attacks returned, so she quickly resumed her good habits and again improved.

Try to eat and sleep well and have as regular a lifestyle as possible.

I've heard many other stories of panic attacks induced by lack of sleep. Once you are a panic attack patient, you have to take very good care of yourself. Sloppy habits that you might have developed when you were well must be eliminated, and better habits of good sleep and good diet need to be developed. One must dedicate oneself to getting better by taking care of oneself. It's not self-indulgence to go to sleep at the same time every night to get eight hours; it's essential behavior.

17. Should I avoid alcohol if I have panic disorder?

Sometimes patients find that alcohol triggers panic attacks. On the other hand, other people find that alcohol helps them avoid panic attacks. The idea is to lead as healthy a lifestyle as possible. I had a patient, an alcoholic, who decided to sober up after receiving one too many citations for driving while under the influence (DWI). After he was abstinent for several months, he developed panic disorder. Instead of restarting alcohol, as many people might have done, he consulted me. I gave him an SSRI, fluoxetine, and set up weekly psychotherapy sessions. It took five weeks for his daily panic attacks to stop. Alcohol is received on the same **GABA** receptor sites as the benzodiazepine medications, like Xanax® and Ativan®, which are used to treat panic disorder. Perhaps his overstimulation of these receptors with alcohol for years and then sudden withdrawal of alcohol triggered his panic attacks. Or it is possible that he had panic disorder, but it was masked during his use of alcohol. Whatever the case, he was able to obtain complete relief from panic attacks with fluoxetine and psychotherapy, both of which were better for him than chronic alcohol use. Once he was on an antidepressant, he felt less desire for alcohol as well. Some alcohol use may be possible if a person's medications do not prohibit its use. However, many antidepressants, the most common medications for panic disorder, do not mix with alcohol. You may try a small amount of wine (one half of a glass) after a meal

Gamma Amino-butyric Acid (GABA)

The most abundant central nervous system amino acid that works to inhibit neuronal transmission; they may malfunction in panic disorder.

but not with your medication to see how you react. If you become drunk very quickly, as some people do, you should not try any more. However, if you notice little or no effect, you may take this small amount a few times per week if you wish. If you can eliminate alcohol completely when taking Ativan® or any other benzodiazepine, that would be preferable.

18. I heard that women get panic attacks more frequently than men. Is that true?

The ratio of women to men is 2:1 in panic disorder without agoraphobia and 3:1 in panic disorder with agoraphobia, but the reason is unknown. Perhaps it's due to a different hormonal influence on the brain. Of course, even though men are in the minority in this condition, many men still suffer from it. Men may also report panic attacks less frequently and try to "tough it out" by drinking or drugging. One of my patients didn't realize he had panic attacks until he stopped his daily use of marijuana. Then he started having them three times a week. In some communities, for example, the Amish in Pennsylvania, where men do not use alcohol or drugs, the ratio of men to women with panic attacks is more even. Perhaps substances like alcohol and drugs mask panic disorder. It is often thought of as a "female problem" that men are reluctant to admit they have.

19. Do African American, Caucasian, Hispanic, Asian, Native American, or any other ethnic groups have panic attacks more frequently than others?

No ethnic group has more panic attacks than any other. However, some groups report panic attacks more frequently, and other groups deny or ignore their significance. A "stiff upper lip" type of coping attitude may be more prevalent in those of Northern European descent and most of our American culture, whereas in Southern Europe, Africa, and South America, people may more easily admit to emotional problems. In Asia, having a mental disorder may lead to ostracism and, in earlier times, some mental patients were locked in the attic or in closets. Such abuse and attitudes certainly would not encourage people to acknowledge that they have panic attacks. In our own North American culture, panic attacks are considered strange, and patients would rather that other people didn't know they are having them.

Different ethnic groups do have different reactions to medications.

Different ethnic groups do have different reactions to medications. For example, Asians tend to need smaller amounts of medications than whites. Perhaps their **p450** liver enzyme systems are not as active. Whatever the reason, Asians may get more side effects or even toxicity from amounts that are considered low or standard by other ethnic groups. Doctors need to be aware and adjust dosages accordingly. Doctors also need to be aware of the differences in reporting among various ethnic groups and to question patients closely if the patient is a member of a culture that minimizes mental disorders. The information may have to be obtained indirectly through other doctors, friends, or relatives.

p450

An enzyme system in the liver, which helps to break down various medicines and foods during metabolism.

20. Is a person's age a factor?

Indeed, age is a factor. Usually people will have panic attacks by their late adolescence to mid-30s. For those who are older, the cause may be medical such as hyperthyroidism or hypoglycemia. There have been several cases of late onset panic attacks. One patient of mine did not have them until he reached his mid-50s. As usual, everyone was concerned that a man of his age had heart disease. He went through a thorough work-up by his cardiologist, including electrocardiogram (EKG), **echocardiogram**, blood tests, among other tests. All of the tests were normal. He was a panic attack patient and was successfully treated with 10 mg Lexapro® once per day, which he continued to take for one year. He was one of the fortunate patients to be able to stop his medicine after that year and be free from panic attacks, at least during the two-year follow-up period for which I treated him. Another of my patients was 70 years old at the time of diagnosis. She had major depression and fears of going outside. When I sat down with her and took a thorough history, I discovered that she also had panic attacks. They would wake her out of sleep in the early morning. She described them as heart palpitations, heavy breathing, and dreadful fear. I told her she had panic attacks and promised that she could be rid of them and her depression with one medication, Zoloft®. After four weeks of 50 mg/day she was relieved of both problems.

Echocardiogram

An ultrasound record of the heart.

Marvin's comments:

I was past my mid-30s when I had my first panic attack, 38 to be exact. I was checked out medically with an EKG, stress test, echocardiogram, and blood tests. Everything was normal.

21. Is there any gene test or blood test that I can take to tell me if I'm at risk for panic attacks?

Currently, there is no blood test or other test that can determine the risk of a person having a panic attack. Your psychiatrist will order blood tests, which include a chemical screen, thyroid function tests, and a complete blood count, to rule out other medical disorders. However, these blood tests cannot determine if you have or will have panic disorder. There is no genetic test at the present time to determine panic attack risk either. The diagnosis is made by clinical observation by your psychiatrist or psychologist. Blood tests of liver and kidney functions can reveal if your body can handle medications. Once we know your tests are within normal limits, we can administer medicines. It is important to obtain these blood tests before or shortly after you start treatment. One patient of mine who had a bad liver due to a prior hepatitis C infection took an antidepressant for panic disorder and felt quite ill. I lowered his dose and he felt much better. A blood test before medication usage would have helped him avoid the problem.

Blood tests cannot determine if you have or will have panic disorder.

22. I heard that eating chocolate or a lot of sugar can cause panic attacks. Is this true?

There are no definitive studies showing that eating chocolate, sugar, or junk foods causes attacks. A good diet is invaluable, of course, in overcoming any sort of illness. When a person begins antidepressant treatment, he or she needs to eat correctly so that weight gain may be kept to a minimum. Recent studies show that dark chocolate in particular is as good for the heart as red wine. So don't feel guilty about eating chocolate. The main idea is that indulging in sugar should be kept to moderate levels, especially if you have diabetes. There are some case reports showing that people who ate sugar excessively are more subject to panic attacks. This is not proven. To understand what a proper diet is, you may consult a nutritionist. Try to avoid the latest fads promoting all protein or all carbohydrates (carbs). The Food and Drug Administration (FDA) provides a pyramidal chart that indicates the right proportion of protein to carbohydrates to fat.

23. I have mitral valve prolapse. Did that cause my panic attacks?

It didn't cause it, but 50% of patients with **mitral valve prolapse (MVP)** also have panic attacks. This condition, in which the bicuspid valve located on the left side of the heart has an excessive backwards movement into the left atrium during contraction of the heart, is associated with panic disorder. The reason the two conditions are associated is not presently known. People with MVP are often aware of their hearts beating and of palpitations, which usually frighten them. MVP is considered a benign condition. It is necessary to take antibiotics **prophylactically** before dental or other procedures, but otherwise it can be ignored. Panic attack patients must learn to ignore or minimize sensations in their bodies. Just because you feel it doesn't mean it's of medical significance. Panic attack patients believe that anything they feel must be abnormal, so they become easily frightened.

Mitral valve prolapse (MVP)

Excessive backwards movement of the mitral valve leaflets into the left atrium of the heart during ventricular systole, sometimes giving mitral regurgitation; MVP has been associated with panic attacks.

Prophylactic

Prevention of a disease or process that can lead to a disease.

24. Once I moved out of the city and into the country I found that my panic attacks stopped. Does relocation make a difference?

Some people find that a city jars their nerves and increases their episodes of panic attacks. I had a patient who lived in the middle of New York City. Her sleep was disturbed by noisy neighbors, car horns, sirens, and buses and trucks careening down her street at all hours. She moved to Woodstock and found that her panic attacks per month were reduced from three to one. It is difficult to tell if the reduction in panic attacks was due to her move to quieter surroundings or if her medication (Zoloft®) was responsible for the improvement. I would say that both the medication and her new surroundings helped her. When many factors are involved in an individual's recovery, it is confusing and often not possible to pinpoint a single cause. Moving to a more rural area reduced the stress on her nervous system and her noradrenergic nerves (the "fight or flight" ones). Living in New York City inevitably stimulates the noradrenergic system and is more activating to the locus ceruleus. Anything that would reduce activity in those areas would be of help. I've had other patients, however, who moved out of the city and felt even more nervous. Panic attack patients should search for whatever decreases their stress levels. Yoga, Pilates exercises, and Alexander techniques are recommended for those who can't change their household location.

Marvin's comments:

Once I moved out of New York City, I felt much better, too. The constant stressors of noise, pollution, and everyone rushing around took a toll on me that I wasn't even aware of. I bought a house in upstate New York and immediately began to enjoy the quiet, fresh air, and leisurely pace. Now I go into my backyard, meditate, and do Tai Chi exercises. I don't want my panic attacks to ever come back. I think I was suppressing a lot of my anxiety in order to live in the city. My dog feels better also. The only thing I regret is having to drive everywhere, but the panic attacks are not a threat anymore, so driving is less of a problem.

25. Can psychotherapy stop panic attacks?

Psychotherapy may help to calm the central nervous system (CNS; See Table 4 and Question 54 for explanations of the different types of therapy.) Tests have shown that many chemicals in the body that relate to stress, such as cortisol levels, are reduced after most types of psychotherapy. If these chemicals are reduced, then panic attacks are reduced. Therapy allows people to deal with their conflicts, feel their feelings, and analyze their behavior patterns. All of these lead to a decrease in panic attacks. Many patients with panic disorder first come into therapy unaware that they are in conflict. They are surprised to learn that they are really quite angry at their boss, sad at the loss of their father, or anxious about their futures. Psychotherapy allows them to identify these feelings, which is unnatural in our North American society. Instead, we are encouraged to suppress most feelings and go about our business. It is the suppression of those feelings that unbalance certain individuals, triggering panic attacks. Also, during psychotherapy, patients can recognize harmful behavioral patterns they may have. For example, Judith, a patient of mine, always sized up everyone sitting in her row in the theatre to make sure that no one seemed hostile to her. If she detected (or imagined) the least bit of hostility on someone's part, she would feel panicky and usually leave the theatre before the show started. She was unaware of this pattern until we discussed it. I suggested that she not check out the people in her row, but rather just ignore them and go into her seat. At first, this was difficult for her because she was so used to automatically assessing people. After much concentration on the subject and practice not doing this, she was able to stop checking everyone out and just take her seat. This decreased her panic attacks. Analysis of other situations in her life also led her to a lessening of anxiety. As a very young child she was subject to the constant scrutiny of her parents because she was the only child. They were overly concerned with her welfare, so she was also. Unconsciously, they were hostile to her because they were older and she occupied so much of their time and energy. They could hardly deal with her youthful exuberance and hyperactivity. Yet, how could they express any of this resentment when they were also feeling so happy to have a child?

Another patient, Ann, felt anxious and would often become panic stricken as she drove in her car. When she stopped at a red light, she believed that the other motorists behind her were impatient at her back and ready to honk in a moment. This made her feel anxious and step on the gas to move the car out of position more quickly then she should have. One time she pulled out before looking and almost had an accident. As we analyzed this situation together, we realized that Ann had negative transference to the motorists behind her. They unconsciously reminded her of her feelings towards her mother, who was constantly on her back, urging her to do things she wasn't ready to do. Ann actually felt anger towards her mother as well as the motorists behind her, but she wasn't able to admit to her feelings until we talked about it. Once Ann understood what she was feeling and was able to express it, then she could feel her anger at the drivers behind her in traffic and hold her position until she was ready to move forward safely after the stoplight changed to green. Her panic attacks diminished as well.

PART THREE

Diagnosis

Are panic attacks related to other illnesses?

Are panic attacks related to depression?

Is it possible to have manic depression and panic disorder?

More . . .

26. Are panic attacks related to other illnesses?

Many illnesses may mimic the symptoms of panic attacks.

Hyperthyroidism

May be enlargement of the thyroid gland and overproduction of thyroid hormones causing nervousness, irritability, and even panicky feelings.

Hyper- or hypoglycemia

Too much or too little sugar in the blood, respectively.

Pheochromo-cytoma

A very rare condition where the hypertensive patient has a benign tumor of the medulla of the adrenal gland; the patient produces a lot of adrenaline or epinephrine, which raises the blood pressure and causes palpitations and sweating, symptoms that make a person believe he or she is having panic attacks.

Many illnesses may mimic the symptoms of panic attacks. For instance, if someone is hyperthyroid, which is when the thyroid gland may be enlarged and produce too many thyroid hormones, the person may be extremely nervous, irritable, and even feel panicky. This person would have to be treated by an endocrinologist, who would be able to determine **hyperthyroidism** by blood tests and at least a physical exam. Another person who thinks she has panic disorder may actually have **hyperglycemia** or **hypoglycemia** (too much or too little sugar in the blood, respectively) that may cause panic attacks. **Pheochromocytoma** may also cause panic attacks. Pheochromocytoma is a condition where the patient has a benign tumor of the medulla of the adrenal gland. This is a very rare condition—fewer than 0.1% of hypertensive patients have it. One of the first symptoms is hypertension because the patients produce a lot of adrenaline or epinephrine, which raises the blood pressure and causes palpitations and sweating. These symptoms make people believe they are having panic attacks.

Thus, it is important that a psychiatrist, who is a medical doctor and can order blood and other diagnostic tests, evaluate the panic attack patient because he or she will be able to rule out other medical illnesses. Psychologists or social workers may treat panic attack patients, but because they are not trained medically, they would not be able to rule out various medical problems that can masquerade as panic disorder. The psychiatrist can then refer the patient to the appropriate doctor, who may be an endocrinologist, cardiologist, or rheumatologist, among others. Most panic attack patients are in good medical condition, but on the occasion when they are not healthy, they need the proper care with the right doctor.

27. Are panic attacks related to depression?

There seems to be a common inheritance for both panic disorder and major depression. Often one can be the precursor of the other or they can occur at the same time. The good news is that antidepressants can treat both conditions. Psychiatrists have very specific criteria for the type of depression that they call major depression. A person needs to have five or more of the following symptoms for at least two consecutive weeks:

1. depressed mood nearly every day (most of the day)*

2. decreased interest or pleasure in all activities*

3. weight loss or gain

4. increased or decreased sleep

5. agitated or slowed down behavior

6. fatigue or loss of energy

7. feeling worthless or guilty

8. decreased concentration

9. recurrent thoughts of death or suicide plans or an attempt

When a person says she feels depressed, it isn't necessarily major depression unless five or more of the above symptoms occur for at least two weeks. Shorter periods of time do not count as major depression.

---

*Symptom must be present according to the *DSM-IV* criteria.

Marvin's comments:

I became depressed after I realized that I had a sickness. My first symptom was waking up too early. I'd go to bed at my usual time, about 11:30 PM, but I'd be wide awake at 5 AM. I wanted to wake up at 7:30 AM. It wasn't anxiety that was disturbing me. I seemed to have some internal alarm clock that wouldn't let me sleep. My appetite was horrible. I could go for a day with only half of a turkey sandwich whereas before I was a three-meal-a-day man with snacks. My pants became baggy on me. I was tired all the time. I was cranky and blue all day long. In the past I would feel bad for a few hours at a time, but this was a relentless onslaught. For the first time in my life I thought about jumping off a bridge. The antidepressant Celexa® that I used for my panic attacks worked against depression, too.

28. Is it possible to have manic depression and panic disorder?

It is possible to have manic depression (which is termed bipolar disorder in the *DSM-IV*) and panic attacks. **Bipolar disorder** is characterized by feelings of alternating elevated mood or euphoria to depression, behaviors of recklessness to listlessness, and flares that can last from weeks to months. This disorder affects more than 2 million adult Americans, but can be managed with medication.

Many patients with manic depression may also get panic attacks. Bipolar patients should be careful when they use antidepressants to treat panic because they may also be setting themselves up for a manic episode with antidepressant use. Thus, a psychopharmacologist should monitor them.

Bipolar disorder

Characterized by feelings of euphoria to depression, behaviors of recklessness to listlessness, and flares that can last from weeks to months; also called manic depression. This disorder affects more than 2 million adult Americans, but can be managed with medication.

Bipolar disorder consists of major depression alternating with manic or hypomanic episodes. Many bipolar patients report the presence of panic attacks either during their depressions or during the course of their manic episodes. Often patients are so confused or overexcited when they are manic or even hypomanic that they can hardly concentrate on panic attacks. They are usually more aware and disturbed by panic attacks when they are depressed and lethargic. Sometimes the medicines employed in bipolar disorder (besides antidepressants), such as the anticonvulsants Depakote®, Tegretol®, and Topamax®, may be prophylactic against panic attacks, too. Some patients have even found lithium carbonate helpful to stop panic attacks. Lithium carbonate is one of the oldest medicines used to treat bipolar disorder. Many people are familiar with manic depression because they've heard stories about Vincent van Gogh or Virginia Woolf, both of whom had bipolar disorder. Tales of famous people with panic disorder are not as common, perhaps because the stories are not as dramatic or those afflicted can hide it better than those who are bipolar.

29. Is there any time of day when panic attacks occur more frequently?

People may get them at any time of day or night, although it is common for a person to have a panic attack outdoors, which may then develop into agoraphobia (see Question 13). Agoraphobia is the fear of going outside or into a place where a person might get a panic attack. Most people who have agoraphobia have panic attacks. One of the prime reasons for a person to seek treatment as quickly as possible for panic disorder is so that agoraphobia does not develop.

Some people are even awakened from sleep at night by panic attacks. This type of panic attack is the most frightening. This type of attack must be distinguished from sleep terror disorder. In **sleep terror disorder**, a patient is often abruptly awakened from sleep with a panicky scream. He or she has intense fear, a rapid heartbeat, deep breathing, and sweating. The person is unresponsive to others trying to comfort him or her and usually has amnesia for the episode. The symptoms of fear—a rapid heartbeat, deep breathing, and sweating—are similar to those with a panic attack, but the unresponsiveness to comfort and amnesia are unique to sleep terror disorder. Panic attack patients are very responsive to comforting, and they always remember their panic attacks and worry about them. If you are awakened from sleep by a panic attack and you're already on medication, your medication is not working adequately. You should inform your treating psychiatrist. Probably, you will need more of the same medicine. Sometimes a tiny addition of 5 mg or so can send a patient into a panic attack-free state. Many times patients or even doctors themselves will be hesitant to change (titrate) a medicine dosage up or down. This is a mistake. Often medicines have to be increased, decreased, or completely changed. Sometimes other medicines are added. For example, I had a patient who was doing well (panic attack-free) on 10 mg of Lexapro®, an antidepressant, for six months. For no reason that we could discern, she started having panic attacks again. I increased her antidepressant to 15 mg and then she was fine for another six months. After that panic attacks returned, so we had to add Topamax® at 25 mg before she was relieved of the panic attacks again. Treatment is an ongoing process, which is why you should visit your doctor at least four times per year.

Sleep terror disorder

Characterized by abruptly waking from sleep with a panicky scream, feelings of intense fear, a rapid heartbeat, deep breathing, and sweating; the person is unresponsive to others trying to comfort him or her and usually has amnesia for the episode. The symptoms of fear— a rapid heartbeat, deep breathing, and sweating—are similar to those with a panic attack, but the unresponsiveness to comfort and amnesia are unique to sleep terror disorder.

If you are awakened from sleep by a panic attack and you're already on medication, your medication is not working adequately.

30. Every time I have to speak in public, I have a panic attack. Does this mean I have panic disorder or social phobia?

You may have both, but if you're more concerned about the panic attack than about public speaking, an argument may be made for panic disorder, but if it's vice versa, then it's social phobia. **Social phobia** is a marked and persistent fear of one or more social or performance situations in which you are exposed to unfamiliar people or to possible scrutiny by others. You fear that you will act in an anxious way that will embarrass or humiliate you. Anytime you are exposed to the feared situation you will have anxiety, which may take the form of a panic attack. Usually you realize your fears and avoid the situations, behaviors that interfere with your social life. Social phobia is common, occurring in 3% to 13% of people. Most people with it fear public speaking more than speaking to strangers or meeting new people. Some fear eating, drinking, or writing in public or using a public restroom. Typically, social phobia starts in the teen years, after a person has been a shy child. Things may start with a humiliating experience and proceed from there. Social phobia can stop you from dating, marrying, and leading a social life. Psychotherapy plus SSRIs and other medications can be used to treat the condition. One patient whom I was treating for panic attacks told me how she was able to speak in front of her English class for the first time without fear once she was on 50 mg of Zoloft®. She also had less trouble talking to men and overcoming her shyness on dates.

Social phobia

A marked and persistent fear of one or more social or performance situations, exposure to unfamiliar people or to possible scrutiny by others. The fear is that the person will act in an anxious way that will be embarrassing or humiliating.

Marvin's comments:

I don't do well with public speaking. This has been a problem since childhood. I remember standing up in front of the classroom, sweating and my mind going blank, and I imagined that the other kids were making fun of me. Maybe there was some truth to this because one time I heard them laughing and felt a rubber band sting my leg while I was fumbling for words. At work I would try to bow out of presentations, too. Once I started taking Celexa®, I found that it helped my social phobia, panic attacks, and depression. One medicine did all that for me. I'm never going to be the kind of guy who volunteers to give a speech, but that is much easier for me now.

31. How is my panic attack different from generalized anxiety disorder, which I also have?

Generalized anxiety disorder (GAD)

A constant, excessive worry with restlessness, fatigue, irritability, and sleep disturbances. GAD patients can also experience their minds going blank, muscle tension, and feeling on edge.

Panic attack anxiety is more intermittent and episodic than **generalized anxiety disorder (GAD)**, which is constant excessive worry with restlessness, fatigue, irritability, and sleep disturbances. GAD patients also can experience their minds going blank, muscle tension, and feeling on edge. Their anxiety is not just focused on having panic attacks (like panic attack patients), being embarrassed in public (like those who have social phobia), or being contaminated (as in patients with obsessive-compulsive disorder). These anxieties cause clinically significant impairment in the social, occupational, or other important areas of functioning. Many GAD patients have an onset of symptoms starting in childhood. SSRIs are often not as effective in treating GAD as they are in panic disorder. Benzodiazepines work well in both disorders, but they are more problematic medicines because of addictions that arise with their use. GAD patients find psychotherapy very helpful, and they should engage in individual treatment as soon as possible.

32. If my panic attack is triggered by fear of heights, is it a panic attack?

There are three kinds of panic attacks:

1. *Unexpected (uncued)*: Panic attacks that occur "out of the blue" and have no triggers associated with them. Many patients complain of these.

2. *Situationally bound (cued)*: A panic attack that occurs after a trigger, like heights, or animals such as dogs or cats.

3. *Situationally predisposed*: A panic attack that may or may not occur after a trigger, where it is likely that one could happen, but it doesn't have to happen.

A panic attack triggered by fear of heights would be considered situationally bound (#2). If your panic attacks always occur after you are exposed to heights and no other times, you may very well become phobic of heights and avoid them. Most people do not have such specific triggers. They are more likely to fall into the first category where the panic attack occurs out of the blue. This is considered more insidious, since the patient can't protect him/herself from a specific situation, like in #2 or #3. Instead, the person becomes fearful of many different situations and may develop agoraphobia.

The third category, situationally predisposed, is present when someone who is afraid of heights is in an apartment on the 30th floor of a high-rise building. It is likely that this person will get a panic attack if someone forces her out on the terrace and she looks down, but she may not get a panic attack just by being in the apartment. It isn't certain that a panic attack will happen every time.

33. After September 11, 2001 I started to have panic attacks on a daily basis. How do I know if I have posttraumatic stress disorder or panic disorder?

Posttraumatic stress disorder (PTSD)

Intense fear, helplessness, or horror after a traumatic event, manifested in persistent, vivid recollections and physical symptoms.

Comorbid

When two disorders exist at the same time.

A person may have both **posttraumatic stress disorder (PTSD)** and panic disorder. A catastrophe like September 11 can trigger panic attacks. If the panic attacks are induced by stimuli recalling the event, such as walking past "ground zero," where the event occurred, then PTSD may be considered a primary diagnosis, or we may say that they are "**comorbid**," that is, the two disorders exist at the same time. The patient with PTSD must have first been exposed to a traumatic event (like 9/11) in which he or she felt threatened by death or serious injury to the physical integrity of self or others. The person's response must involve intense fear, helplessness, or horror. Afterwards, the traumatic event is persistently re-experienced by distressing recollections, dreams, flashbacks, and psychological distress to internal and/or external cues that represent the traumatic event. Also, a PTSD patient must have a physiological reactivity when re-exposed to things surrounding the event (like sweating or rapid heart rate). The PTSD victim avoids the stimuli associated with the trauma, has feelings of detachment, a sense of a foreshortened future, and a restricted range of emotions. Increased arousal causes hypervigilance, anger, and sleep problems. A patient of mine who was raped had a panic attack every time she saw a movie or a TV program where another woman was raped. She would also have nightmares about her own rape if she saw a rape in the movies or on TV. The more she worked on the issues the rape brought up for her, the more relieved of panic attacks and, finally, the better she felt.

34. When my husband was taken to the emergency room after having a panic attack (we mistakenly thought it was a heart attack), he was found to have a fast heart rate and high BP. Yet, the doctors ignored that and told him he only had panic disorder. Should we be concerned?

Many times people think they are having a heart attack until the emergency room doctor or a cardiologist rules out heart disease, and a diagnosis of panic disorder is made. A fast heart rate and high blood pressure (BP) may occur during panic attacks without indicating heart problems. If these two symptoms clear up and are not present usually, there is no need for concern. You should concentrate on trying to treat the panic disorder.

The first step is to consult a psychiatrist, who will probably recommend that your husband start taking an anxiolytic and an antidepressant. In many instances, psychotherapy will be recommended as well. Sometimes patients don't believe that they are physically well. They go from doctor to doctor seeking relief from some imaginary physical illness. Once panic attacks are stopped, your husband will be able to resume a normal life. **Hypochondriasis**, a condition where one believes and worries that one is ill when one is not, is not a good state to be in if one is also a panic attack patient. Worrying about some non-existent medical condition can trigger a panic attack and vice versa, a panic attack can trigger excessive concern about the heart, blood pressure, or lungs.

Hypochondriasis

A condition where one believes and worries that one is ill when one is not.

35. After getting panic attacks I became discouraged and ashamed of myself. Is this common?

Feelings of shame and discouragement after a panic attack are common.

Depression

A state of lowered mood, usually with disturbances of sleep, appetite, suicidal thoughts, etc.

Unfortunately, feelings of shame and discouragement after a panic attack are common. A psychiatrist should consult with you to determine if you also have depression, which commonly occurs with panic disorder. The rate may be higher than 50% (see Question 27). Signs of **depression** are depressed mood nearly every day for two weeks, decreased pleasure in activities, weight loss or gain, insomnia or hypersomnia, agitation or psychomotor retardation, fatigue, guilt, decreased concentration, and suicidal ideation (having thoughts of killing yourself). Discouragement occurs when we have unreal expectations for ourselves. For example, if we believe that we will be immune from disease, we are living in a fantasy. Many times people are "trained" to believe that nothing negative can ever happen to them. The "training" is an unconscious process done by parents and other caretakers who have all good intentions. The problem is that if we don't have mental room for sickness and untoward events, we are unprepared for the natural course of events, which inevitably include negative experiences.

People often become discouraged when any kind of disorder is diagnosed and they find it difficult to adapt. Psychotherapy is helpful, because it enables us to retrain ourselves to accept the natural course of events. Our discouragement is decreased if we can understand where panic disorder and other sicknesses fit into the scheme of life.

A patient of mine did very well in her life in terms of a career, marriage, and children until she started having panic attacks at age 40. This is a late onset for this disorder, but it does happen more often than we think. At that point, she became very discouraged and believed her good fortune was over. She believed that now she would have only bad luck and a downward course to her life. She came to me for psychotherapy only because she didn't know what else she could do. She was against medication. I had to work hard to convince her to take an SSRI to get rid of her panic attacks. That was the first hurdle. She was amazed that she was able to be panic attack-free after four weeks on Celexa®. She still believed that she was destined for a horrible second part to her life. The second hurdle was to examine her negative mindset, which she merely assumed was normal given her circumstances. I asked her to come to sessions three times per week, which she did. She was surprised to see how well she felt after medicine and therapy, and her shame decreased.

PART FOUR

Prevention and Treatment

What kind of doctor treats panic attacks?

I heard it wasn't a good idea to take Valium® or Xanax® to deal with panic attacks. What are these drugs?

What medicines should be taken to stop panic attacks?

More . . .

36. What kind of doctor treats panic attacks?

A **psychiatrist**, a medical doctor specializing in psychiatry, is the medical expert who treats panic attacks. This doctor may prescribe medications and do psychotherapy. **Behavioral therapy** is sometimes effective in treating panic disorder. It focuses on changing overt behavior by a variety of techniques (systematic desensitization, relaxation training, flooding, participant modeling, and positive and negative reinforcement (see Question 41). A **psychologist** (PhD in psychology) or a **social worker** (LCSW or CSW) may administer behavioral treatment or do other kinds of psychotherapy as well as a psychiatrist, but neither can prescribe medications. Many times people mix up a psychiatrist and a psychologist. The difference is great. A "therapist" *per se* does not indicate anything about the person's education and qualifications, because he or she may be a psychiatrist, psychologist, social worker, minister, rabbi, nurse, or lay person (someone without a degree), all of whom have varying degrees of expertise. A psychiatrist is the only kind of medical doctor one should entrust with medications for panic attacks. A psychiatrist may have an M.D. (doctor of medicine) or D.O. (a doctor of osteopathic medicine) degree. M.D.s and D.O.s are the only two types of complete physicians in the United States. This means that all must have completed a degree program in medicine after graduating from a college or university and then passed a state medical board examination to obtain a license to practice. These medical doctors can be board-certified in psychiatry, meaning they have completed additional study hours in this particular field of medicine, which would be an extra benefit for the patient.

37. I heard it wasn't a good idea to take Valium® or Xanax® to deal with panic attacks. What are these drugs?

Both Valium® and Xanax® are addictive drugs. They are in the category of **benzodiazepines**. These medicines should be used sparingly if at all. One doesn't need to acquire an addiction in addition to panic disorder. Other medicines in this category are Klonopin®, Ativan®, and Librium®. Psychiatrists often give a panic attack patient these medicines at the beginning of treatment to immediately decrease anxiety in the panic attack patient. In the long run they are not the medicines that should be used for panic disorder because they affect the GABA system adversely. The **GABA system** is the gamma-aminobutyric acid system, which consists of neurotransmitters in various parts of the brain that are responsible for inhibiting **neurons**. If the GABA system is not working well, nerve cells are not turned off (inhibited) when they should be and excess stimulation can occur, resulting in panic attacks and other unwanted events. The brain may have its own endogenous benzodiazepines, and one theory claims that panic attack patients don't have enough of these natural substances in their brains. Thus, Valium® and Xanax® should be used sparingly if at all. For example, if a new panic attack patient who is getting three to five attacks per day comes to me begging for immediate relief, I will prescribe 0.5 mg of Xanax® to be taken two to three times per day along with an SSRI like Zoloft®. We have to wait three to four weeks for the Zoloft® to kick in, but in the meantime, she can obtain relief with Xanax®.

Benzodiazepines

A type of drug used for short-term treatment of panic attacks to decrease anxiety and depression; potentially addictive.

GABA system

The system of neurotransmitters in various parts of the brain that are responsible for inhibiting neurons. If the GABA system is not working well, nerve cells are not turned off (inhibited) when they should be, and excess stimulation can occur that results in panic attacks and other unwanted events.

Neuron

A nerve cell, the basic cell unit of the brain and spinal cord.

Antidepressants

The best medicines to stop panic attacks; nonaddictive and may benefit the nervous system in many ways.

Selective serotonin reuptake inhibitors (SSRIs)

A type of antidepressant that doesn't allow serotonin to be taken up again by neuroreceptors, thereby causing more serotonin to be present to the neurons, which decreases panic attacks; includes drugs such as Prozac®, Zoloft®, Paxil®, Celexa®, Luvox®, and Lexapro®.

Serotonin

A neurotransmitter that may be decreased in depression and panic attacks.

Tricylic antidepressants (TCAs)

Medications that provide more norepinephrine at important receptor sites in the brain; includes Tofranil® and Norpramin®.

Receptor

A protein molecule on the surface of a cell that receives and binds neurotransmitters, hormones, etc.

Psychopharmacologist

Psychiatrist who specializes in prescribing medicines for mental disorders.

38. What medicines should be taken to stop panic attacks?

Antidepressants are the best medicines to stop panic attacks (**Table 2**). They are nonaddictive and may benefit the nervous system in many ways. The **selective serotonin reuptake inhibitors (SSRIs)** allow more **serotonin** to be present to the neurons and thus, decrease panic attacks. These medicines include Prozac®, Zoloft®, Paxil®, Celexa®, Luvox®, and Lexapro®. Other variants like Effexor® are useful, too. The older **tricylic antidepressants (TCAs)** such as Tofranil® and Norpramin® are effective as well. These TCAs provide more norepinephrine at important **receptor** sites in the brain. Benzodiazepines, which are addictive tranquilizers, may be used parsimoniously, if at all. These include medicines like Ativan® and Xanax® (see Question 37). Sometimes the psychiatrist may prescribe these addictive medicines along with an antidepressant at the beginning of treatment until the antidepressant has time to work. Most antidepressants take from two to six weeks to "kick in," so an adjunct like Xanax® may be necessary. Once the antidepressant is working, the benzodiazepine, such as Xanax®, can be slowly discontinued. If a patient tries to stop taking Xanax® too quickly, it could result in a convulsion. Therefore, it is important to consult your **psychopharmacologist**, the psychiatrist who specializes in prescribing medicines for mental disorders, before stopping or starting any medicines for mental disorders. There is no reason to fear medication if you are under a competent doctor's care. Somehow medications have acquired a bad reputation and patients believe they should try everything they can to stay way from medicine. They want to try "natural ways" of treating panic disorders. Natural things are fine if they work, but often they don't work for mental disorders.

Table 2 Medicines Used for Panic Disorders

Drug	Dosage
Antidepressants	
Selective-serotonin-reuptake-inhibitors (SSRIs)	
Escitalopram (Lexapro®)	5–20 mg/day
Citalopram (Celexa®)	10–30 mg/day
Fluoxetine (Prozac®)	5–20 mg/day
Paroxetine (Paxil®)	10–30 mg/day
Sertraline (Zoloft®)	25–100 mg/day
Fluvoxamine (Luvox®)	50-300 mg/day
TCAs	
Imipramine (Tofranil®)	50–100 mg/day
Nortriptyline (Pamelor®)	50–100 mg/day
Desipramine (Norpramin®)	50–100 mg/day
MAOIs	
Tranylcypromine (Parnate®)	10-20 mg/day
Phenelzine (Nardil®)	15-45 mg/day
Others	
Venlafaxine (Effexor®)	37.5–150 mg/day
Mirtazapine (Remeron®)	45–60 mg/day
Duloxetine (Cymbalta®)	30-60 mg/day
Minor Tranquilizers (Benzodiazepines)	
Long-Acting	
Clonazepam (Klonopin®)	0.5–2 mg/day
Diazepam (Valium®)	2–5 mg/day
Short-Acting	
Alprazolam (Xanax®)	0.25–2 mg four times/day
Lorazepam (Ativan®)	0.5 mg–2 mg two times/day

Nature produces many substances that people can exploit. For instance, during medieval times monks grew foxglove flowers for beauty. But one day they discovered that an essence of the flower (after distillation) given to patients with bad hearts helped them to function better. What they were using was basically the medicine digitalis. Nowadays, digitalis is used all the time for chronic heart failure patients, but we don't need to distill it from foxglove flowers. It can be produced artificially. This is done with most medicines; they may have started as natural remedies that ended up as artificial medications. Some herbalists argue that the plant contains other parts that shouldn't be omitted, but for mass production and economic reasons, we manufacture the plants' chemicals.

Marvin's comments:

Right now I'm taking Celexa®, which is one of the SSRIs Dr. Berman talks about. We tried Prozac® at first, but I felt too nervous and it was hard to sleep. Then we tried Zoloft®. I didn't find much help from it, even though I took up to 150 mg. I always felt nauseous and dizzy with Zoloft® and it didn't take the panic attacks completely away. Celexa® worked after only two weeks. I need just 10 mg per day and I don't have side effects.

39. When I started to take 25 mg of Zoloft® each day for my panic attacks, I became nauseous and had a bad headache. Does this mean I can't use this medicine?

Experiencing nausea and headaches after taking an antidepressant does not mean that you can't take it. Many times panic attack patients are very sensitive to SSRIs like Zoloft® (see Question 38). The doctor will prescribe a very low dose and gradually increase the amount until the patient's body can tolerate the dosage that is right for him or her. The usual dosage of Zoloft® for a panic disorder patient is 25 to 75 mg. Some people need smaller doses and some much larger. The amount of medicine is not just proportional to body weight, but it is also dependent on a person's liver function. SSRIs can cause nausea because they interact with the serotonin receptors in the gastrointestinal tract. Eventually one becomes accustomed to these medicines and can tolerate them. Eating dry soda crackers or drinking ginger ale with the medicine may help. Headaches also can be a problem at the beginning of treatment, although in the long run SSRIs may be prophylactic against migraines. The main idea is to try to remain calm and not overreact to each side effect. There is such a thing as a **nocebo reaction**. This is the opposite of a **placebo reaction** where a person has a positive effect from a sugar pill. In the nocebo effect, a patient feels frightened of a medicine and so has a bad reaction to an innocuous substance. These bad reactions may be nausea, headaches, shakiness, diarrhea, etc. It is best to work closely with your psychiatrist to avoid these problems. For headaches, Tylenol® and **nonsteroidal anti-inflammatory drugs (NSAIDs)** are useful. Nausea is a frequent side effect at the beginning of treatment. The idea is to try to stay on the prescribed medicines long enough for them to kick in and take effect.

Marvin's comments:

I was sensitive to Zoloft®, too. I used to get migraine headaches that were so bad that it was like someone sticking a knife over my left eyebrow. I'd have to take aspirin and lie down in a dark room until they worked. Celexa® actually took my headaches away. I'm happy with this medicine. I don't mind if I have to use it for the rest of my life. Dr. Berman wanted to switch me to some other medicine, Lexapro®, that she said

Nocebo reaction

A reaction in which a patient feels frightened of a medicine and so has a bad reaction to an innocuous substance.

Placebo reaction

A reaction in which a person has a positive effect from an innocuous substance such as a sugar pill.

Nonsteroidal anti-inflammatory drugs (NSAIDs)

A large number of drugs exerting an active effect to reduce or eliminate inflammation (sometimes analgesic and antipyretic actions, too); examples include: aspirin, ibuprofen, indomethacine, and naproxen.

was related to Celexa®, but I figured, why change things if they're working well? Just because you have a bad reaction to something at the beginning, it doesn't mean you won't be able to use it later. Trust your doctor and try to work with him or her.

40. Why are some people cured of panic attacks and some not cured?

It's not clear why some people take medicines and then never have another panic attack, and why others are subject to panic attacks indefinitely. The ratio between them is thought to be about 50/50. This means that 50% who take antidepressants for panic attacks may never have another one after one year of treatment, and 50% will get reoccurrences. The best plan is to attempt to take medication for a year before discontinuing. I have found that when patients attempt to stop medication earlier than one year, their episodes of panic attacks recur. Doing psychotherapy while taking medication is one of the best treatment plans. Psychotherapy can actually change the chemistry of the brain. We know that it works on both a physical and emotional level. If you can learn to modify your responses to frightening internal stimuli—like in a panic attack—you are better able to cope with panic disorder.

Psychotherapy can actually change the chemistry of the brain.

41. What is behavioral therapy, and how does it work?

Behavioral therapy is an application of learning principles to the treatment of behavioral disorders. In the 1960s, behavioral treatment began to be employed with a goal of modifying maladaptive behavior into new, non-anxiety-provoking behavior patterns. The techniques include: systematic desensitization, relaxation training, flooding, aversion participant modeling, positive and negative reinforcement, and biofeedback. The idea is that negative behaviors have been conditioned, so treatment consists of re-conditioning. **Conditioning** is the process of acquiring, developing, educating, establishing, learning, or training new responses in an individual. When the triggers of a panic attack are identified, those events that cause an automatic response, behavioral therapy can help to unlink those triggers.

Conditioning

The process of acquiring, developing, educating, establishing, learning, or training new responses in an individual.

If a woman always has panic attacks on a bus, the behavioral therapist will try to replace her muscle tenseness, shallow breathing, and fear images with muscle relaxation, deep breathing, and peaceful images while she rides the bus. Depending on the individual and how the techniques are practiced, these techniques can be quite effective. They are especially useful for treating specific phobias, such as agoraphobia (irrational fear of going outside or leaving the familiar settings of a home), animal phobias, and hydrophobia (fear of water). Panic attack patients can be taught to disregard many of the bodily sensations of which they are hyperaware, for example, heart palpitations and tingling in the arms and legs. Instead of concentrating on these meaningless feelings, they learn how to breathe deeply and to imagine pleasant things if a panic attack begins.

Lately, **flooding techniques** have been popular, in which a patient is exposed to his worst fear all at once. For example, if someone is terrified of heights, he'll be taken to the top of the Empire State Building immediately, rather than slowly building up to the trip, as would be done in some of the other behavioral therapy techniques. But flooding would be detrimental to panic attack patients, so it should not be tried.

Flooding technique

A therapy in which a patient is exposed to his worst fear all at once in an effort to lessen or eliminate the fear; not recommended for panic attack patients.

42. What is the worst case of panic attacks you've ever treated?

One time I treated a high school teacher who had panic attacks at least 20 times per day for two years. She would hardly finish one attack before another one would start. They were overwhelming, relentless attacks accompanied by a racing heart, shortness of breath, and a fear of dying or going crazy. She stopped working, driving her car, and was house bound at 45 years old. Her daughter brought her to consult with me. I started her on Ativan® (1 mg four times per day) and Zoloft® (25 mg per day for one week and then 50 mg per day). Over four weeks the rate of her panic attacks diminished to ten per day. She was happy about that. Once the Zoloft® kicked in after a month and a half, her panic attacks leveled off to one every other week. The patient was enormously relieved. She returned to work, started to drive again, and was able to have a normal life once more. Eventually, after several months, her panic attacks stopped. She never wanted to discontinue her medications and so stayed on them to the present time, even though I told her she could try to stop them after one year. Many panic attack patients are dedicated to taking their medicines, especially if they suffered as much as this woman.

43. Once I'm relieved of panic attacks, can they ever return?

Unfortunately, they may return after medication and/or therapy is stopped.[1] In some cases they never return; in others, they return after several years. The good news is that medications and therapy can always be restarted. Stressful situations such as deaths in the family, loss of

---

[1] Sometimes they even return when a patient is on medication.

business, loss of health, cancer scares, car accidents, 9/11 or other terrorist attacks can re-trigger panic disorder. Often patients with panic disorder have a rigid, perfectionist mindset that will not allow for any errors or any illnesses the patient might have. Through insight-oriented psychotherapies, patients can explore the meaning of illness and how to adapt to it. We in the mental health community would like to be able to guarantee no more panic attacks, but we can't do that. Many illnesses are chronic and patients have to adapt to them over the years. This is true for hypertension, diabetes, and arthritis. It is true for many panic attack patients as well.

Table 3 lists some prevention strategies that you may find helpful.

44. I heard that if I took vitamin B supplements I would be able to rid myself of panic attacks. Is that true?

There are no studies proving that vitamin B or any other vitamin supplements would be helpful. Throughout the years one vitamin therapy or another has been promoted

Table 3 Prevention Strategies

1. Avoid caffeine (coffee, teas, cola, etc.).
2. Avoid stimulant medications.
   A. Amphetamines
   B. Ephedra (Ma Huang)
   C. Yohimbine
3. Try to get 6 to 8 hours of sleep/day.
4. Eat a healthy diet with lots of vegetables and fruits.
5. Do not use cocaine.
6. Avoid low oxygen environments like high altitudes.

The best plan is to eat well with three meals per day and a multi-vitamin once a day.

Norepinephrine

A catecholamine hormone stored in the adrenal medulla that is secreted in response to hypotension and physical stress; used pharmacologically as a vasopressor.

as "the cure" for panic disorder. So far, none of them is holding up after research and long clinical trials. The best plan is to eat well with three meals per day and a multivitamin once a day. Good hydration, which means drinking several glasses of water each day, is also important. After dieting, often patients will need less medication because their body weight has declined. It is a good idea to try and reach the optimal body weight for your height. Too much weight may activate the cortisol system and that will trigger negative feedback systems in **norepinephrine**, which may stimulate panic attacks. Many patients will try alternative medicine like acupuncture, herbal treatments, and so forth. Sometimes these therapies help and sometimes they don't. Most M.D.s are not familiar with these other treatment modes and can't answer questions about them.

45. I once had a panic attack during sex. In the back of my mind, I fear having another attack whenever I have sex. How can I relieve this fear?

Behavioral therapy or psychoanalytically oriented treatment might be the best way to help with this problem of linking sex with anxiety. You need to relieve yourself of the fear so you will not become phobic of sex. People become phobic of many activities if they have panic attacks during these activities. The classical ones are sex, driving, being in a theatre, or on a crowded bus or subway. Numerous times I've heard stories of patients becoming phobic of one thing or another. If a panic attack patient is in psychotherapy, he or she can deal with these issues as they arise. If you find yourself shying away from sex because you've had a panic attack at that time, you should ask yourself what your conflicts are with this issue. Perhaps you don't have a conflict, and the two events just happen to coincide with each other. Just because A and B occur one right after the other, it doesn't mean that A caused B. Most people have some guilt about sex because of the way our society views this activity, even if it is between two mutually consenting adults who are married to each other. If there is conflict and guilt, then that can stir up the adrenaline system and a panic attack can occur. It is a good policy to be aware of the feelings behind any activity because sometimes that awareness alone can abort a panic attack. Even activities like being in a crowded bus can stir up hostility, paranoia, and other negative feelings that can trigger panic. Psychotherapy inspires awareness, which can prevent panic attacks.

PART FIVE

Surviving

How can I get my spouse to understand the problem?

I am becoming afraid to go outside because
I am afraid of having a panic attack in public.
What can I do?

Will I pass this condition on to my children?

More . . .

46. I was told not to drink once I started my medicine (Zoloft®) for panic disorder. However, I found if I drank even a small glass of whiskey each night (I took Zoloft® in the AM), I felt better and the one panic attack per week that I was left with cleared up. How can that be?

Alcohol gets into the same receptor sites as Valium®, Ativan®, and Xanax® (benzodiazepines). Like those medicines, alcohol can temporarily make a person feel better, but in the long run, alcohol and even these medicines can lead to addiction and other problems. I had a patient who had been drinking alcohol excessively every day since his teens. Finally at 38, he had one too many DWI citations and decided to stop. His doctor happily monitored his patient's progress. The patient attended Alcoholics Anonymous (AA) meetings and felt virtuous about his abstinence. Then he suddenly was struck with panic attacks while driving. He didn't know what was going on. His doctor, a general practitioner, ran blood tests, an EKG, and so forth on the patient, but he couldn't find anything wrong physically. Finally, the doctor realized that his patient was describing panic attacks and sent the man to me. I placed this patient on 10 mg of Celexa® and within three weeks the panic attacks stopped. We were all pleased with the results. Then one day the patient asked me if he could restart alcohol. Of course, I laughed and said no. He wanted to know if his abstinence had caused the panic attacks. I told him that it might have been that the withdrawal of alcohol, after so many years of use, had triggered an imbalance in the serotonin–norepinephrine–epinephrine system. But not much is known at present about the effects of alcohol on that system. Drinking was the last thing he needed, but his question was, ironically, entirely logical.

47. How can I get my spouse to understand the problem?

Sometimes discussing your panic attacks with a loved one can be difficult. You can explain that your heart is racing, you feel faint, and that you fear you will die. Most spouses or significant others will try to reassure you that everything is O.K. Because they are not experiencing your physical sensations, they may not be able to comprehend or fully relate to your panic attacks. As you understand more about your own condition, you will be able to explain details to them, which will help them to help you. Perhaps you can tell them that it's like being chased by your worst enemy, only the enemy is invisible and thus more frightening. Tell them to hold your hand sometimes and otherwise be available to you as a support system.

I had one patient who couldn't get on the subway unless she held her husband's hand. This helped her to feel better and not have a panic attack. After her medications started working, I encouraged her to leave her husband at home and go alone into the subway. She didn't want to become phobic so she complied, but it was very difficult for her. For the first few times alone, she felt anxious and frightened that she would have a panic attack (she didn't). Too much hand-holding, as in this case, can promote dependency and phobias.

Spouses need to realize that panic attacks are due to a chemical imbalance in the brain and not just random fear. Some spouses may believe that their mates are "faking it" to receive attention. Most likely this is not the case, although a large majority of the public continues to believe so. Positron emission tomography (PET) scans and other tests have shown that epinephrine floods into the brain during panic attacks. Perhaps skeptical spouses can be shown some of these "hard" facts or can visit the psychiatrist with you to gain greater understanding.

48. I am becoming scared of going outside because I am afraid of having a panic attack in public. What can I do?

The fear of having a panic attack in public is a common problem.

The fear of having a panic attack in public is a common problem. People with panic disorder may become agoraphobic (fear of going outside). It is necessary to force yourself outside and to deal with the fears so they don't disable you. You may deal with agoraphobia through medication or behavioral treatment. Some people also become afraid of sitting in theaters, and riding in buses, airplanes, and cars. These fears must be treated quickly so people don't become agoraphobic.

One of my panic attack patients didn't treat her fear of going outside quickly enough and became housebound for six months. She was so overwhelmed by the thought of leaving her familiar surroundings that she wasn't able to get out to work in her office. Instead, she worked at home on her computer. Through e-mail and the Internet, she shopped, socialized, wrote business communications, and so on. Her real world grew smaller and smaller. Occasionally her grown children would visit her, but basically she led an isolated existence. Finally, after five months she consented to having a psychologist visit her three times per week. The doctor came into the patient's home and then accompanied her outside for short intervals of time for the first two weeks of treatment. My patient was terrified to go outside, but she was able to do it in the presence of the psychologist. Gradually, their excursions outside grew longer and longer until the patient was able to venture out on her own. The whole process was difficult and expensive, but she conquered her agoraphobia, returned to work, and continued her normal life of going outside whenever she desired. It would have been better if she could have addressed her problem in therapy as it occurred, so she wouldn't have had to endure being housebound for half of a year.

If your job depends on you going outside, you might be forced to tell your boss about your condition. Some bosses may not look kindly upon any mental disorder, but under the Americans with Disabilities Act that was passed into law in 1992, supervisors are required to accommodate any disability in the workplace. Panic disorder with agoraphobia can be quite disabling. I would tell the boss if panic attacks caused you to become housebound.

49. Will I pass this condition on to my children?

A tendency to have panic attacks can be inherited. It's thought that first-degree biological relatives of individuals with panic disorder are eight times more likely to develop panic attacks. If the age of onset is before age 20, then these relatives have up to 20 times the chance to get panic disorder. Twin studies indicate a genetic component.

People are frightened of passing on their illnesses to their children, and we in the medical community are not able to help very much. In the future, there is a strong probability that we will be able to pick out which genes are causing the problem and modify them. Geneticists are working on finding the specific genes that cause psychiatric disorders. In the meantime, however, if you wish to have children, do so; try to provide them with the best environment that you can, which includes reduced stress. If you notice your child struggling with anxiety or panic attacks, please get help for him or her as soon as possible. There are many studies showing that early interventions in many mental disorders help to cut down their severity and the length of the illness. Studies have not been done specifically with panic disorder, but they have been with schizophrenia. It looks as though medications and therapy instituted early enough are of enormous value.

Early inter-ventions in many mental disorders help to cut down their severity.

50. Are there any problems with panic attacks during pregnancy?

Women may get panic attacks during pregnancy or during some part of their menstrual cycles. The difficulty in pregnancy is treatment without disturbing the fetus. Many current studies show that it is O.K. to use antidepressants during pregnancy if it is necessary. However, not introducing extra medicines during the time of pregnancy is often the best policy.

I had a pregnant patient with panic attacks who didn't want to take any medicines. Instead, we tried relaxation techniques whenever she felt a panic attack coming on. She would lie down in a comfortable position, do deep breathing and progressive muscle relaxation, starting at the feet and working up to the top of her head. The panic attacks didn't completely stop with this technique, but they were considerably lessened.

51. Will my panic attacks last for the rest of my life?

The natural course of panic attacks throughout the lifespan has not been officially documented, but it is believed that panic attacks begin somewhere between the late teens and the mid-30s. Some people may have them in early childhood or after age 45. In many individuals, panic attacks may fade out after they reach their 50s. In others, the panic attacks may grow stronger with aging and more stress. Some patients have continuous and severe ones throughout their lives. There is no way to predict who will have what intensity or how often they will occur. According to the *DSM-IV*, follow-up studies have shown that after 6 to 10 years of treatment, 30% are well, 40% to 50% are improved but symptomatic, and 20% to 30% are symptomatic and the same or slightly worse. It is a good idea to have visits with a psychiatrist at least one time per year if you are not taking medicines, and three to four times per year if you are taking medicines.

If you are in psychotherapy, you may attend sessions as often as three times per week or as infrequently as once per month. Basically, panic disorder should be considered a chronic condition that can reoccur with added stress. Like all chronic conditions, there are remissions and exacerbations. I think most patients are less discouraged with everything if they have this long-term perspective.

52. My fiancée is 25 years old. She has panic attacks and is taking Lexapro®, which helps her. What can I expect once we're married? Will panic attacks interfere with pregnancy or childbirth?

Usually medications like Lexapro® or one of the other antidepressants are able to keep panic attacks in check or able to keep people panic-attack free. Once you and your fiancée decide when you want to have children, she should consult with her psychiatrist and see if she can stop medication before she becomes pregnant (see Question 50). It is always better to be as free of medications as possible during pregnancy. However, if she still has panic attacks during the pregnancy, she can take some antidepressants (e.g., Zoloft®), which have been studied and found to be the least dangerous to a fetus, or she can take nothing and just do therapy. Panic attacks won't interfere with pregnancy or childbirth, causing premature abortion on anything like that. The mother will be uncomfortable during a panic attack, but she can learn to relax and comfort herself.

Panic attacks won't interfere with pregnancy or childbirth.

53. My 16-year-old daughter has panic attacks. Does this mean I should discourage her from participation in sports or cheerleading?

In fact, your daughter should be encouraged to try out for various sports and to be as active as possible. Any activity that increases health and outdoor activity would be good for a girl with panic disorder. We want to prevent agoraphobia (fear of the outdoors), which is far too common in panic attack patients. Healthy activities like sports have a positive biochemical feedback on the nervous system, too.

We want to reduce shame and embarrassment. If your daughter continues with her sports and cheerleading, she will have many activities to look forward to. If she starts to feel embarrassed about her condition, she can talk with friends and coaches about her problems. She will increase her self-esteem with these positive activities and prevent self-loathing and recrimination. Shame becomes less available if one is involved in the world and participating well.

54. What kinds of therapies are good for panic attack patients?

Medication therapy (see Question 38) is essential, and cognitive behavioral therapy (see Question 41) has been found to be effective as well. Many studies show that a combination of both treatments works the best. In cognitive behavioral therapy, the patient focuses on his or her false beliefs about panic attacks and tries to correct them with accurate information. Dizziness, for example, is misinterpreted by the panic attack patient as a horrible sign of sickness when it is really nothing. The cognitive therapist allows the patient to consider this false belief and imparts new, correct beliefs about the significance of dizziness.

A patient of mine in her twenties always focused on her rapidly beating heart during a panic attack, which she thought indicated a terrible cardiac condition. Given her age and overall excellent physical condition, I didn't think she had a problem, but I advised her to get a physical exam, blood tests, and an electrocardiogram (EKG) just to be sure. As predicted, she was fine. During therapy sessions, we discovered that her father died from a heart attack when he was in his fifties, and she believed that her rapidly beating heart would cause her to die in the same way, only in her twenties. Once she had evidence from her medical exam that everything was fine, I was able to teach her to hold an idea of her good heath in her thoughts whenever her heart beat rapidly, instead of the idea about her father dying. In this way, she was able to calm herself with positive thoughts. Her negative cognition (or thought) was replaced with a positive cognition. For her, cognitive behavioral therapy was beneficial.

Other patients can use regular psychoanalytical psychotherapy once or twice a week, which consists of exploring any thoughts patients may have about anything that concerns them. Group therapy in which several patients talk about their problems is also helpful. Traditional psychoanalysis on the couch three to four times per week is not recommended because it promotes regression, which is not thought to be that useful. **Table 4** lists the types of psychotherapies and notes whether each is useful for someone who has panic attacks.

Marvin's comments:

Along with my medication, I've been doing individual psychotherapy with a social worker therapist one time per week. Dr. Berman sees me every few months for medication. This plan works well for me. I'm not doing cognitive behavioral therapy but I am doing what's called psychoanalytically oriented psychotherapy. I sit up in a chair and face my therapist. My job is to show up on time, which isn't hard for me, and get in touch with whatever feelings I'm having (which

Table 4 Types of Psychotherapies

Type	Definition	Usefulness for Panic Disorder
Cognitive therapy	Cognition (thoughts) can be analyzed and changed	Very useful
Behavior therapy (including cognitive-behavioral)	Emphasis on behavior and changing it	Useful
Psychoanalytical psychotherapy	Therapy that may be supportive and/or insight-oriented	Very useful
Psychoanalysis	Freudian resolution of childhood neurosis	Not very useful
Group psychotherapy	Several patients treated together to effect personality change	Useful as an adjunct
Brief psychotherapy	Time-limited therapies based on psychoanalysis	Useful
Family therapy	Family members treated together to understand their pattern of interaction	Useful as an adjunct

is hard for me). Before I started therapy (on Dr. Berman's recommendation) I never knew what feelings I was having. The way I understand it, one of the reasons we have panic attacks is that we suppress our feelings and that somehow causes triggering of the faulty alarm system. These days I'm able to identify feelings as I have them, rather than push them underground and watch them overwhelm me at some later date.

55. I feel like I'm having a convulsion when I have a panic attack. Are they related?

A panic attack is not a convulsion, but often patients feel like they are the same. With panic attacks, patients describe a suffocating sensation, racing heart, shaking, and fear of going crazy. Hyperventilation (shallow, rapid breaths) or overbreathing before a seizure may be similar. Patients complain of dizziness, a sense of floating, anxiety, abdominal discomfort, muscle twitches, flushing, and the mind going blank. Prolonged hyperventilation can result in a seizure in a vulnerable individual. People who have **temporal lobe epilepsy**—that is, their epileptic foci are located in the temporal lobe of the brain—often have panic attacks. However, temporal lobe epilepsy patients have abnormal electroencephalograms (EEGs) and the majority of panic attack patients don't.

Temporal lobe epilepsy

A seizure disorder in which epileptic foci are located in the temporal lobe of the brain.

There have been some reports of anticonvulsants like Tegretol®, Depakote®, and Neurontin® helping to control panic attacks. Antidepressants like SSRIs or even TCAs are used more traditionally for panic disorder (see Questions 27 and 38). In some cases these antidepressants might even lower the seizure threshold, so if it were entirely a seizure-like process occurring in the brain during a panic attack, then antidepressants would not help.

56. I have panic attacks while driving. Do you have any suggestions on how to help myself?

Many patients have panic attacks during driving, especially on highways. Perhaps it's because they feel trapped in a car and can't pull off the road so easily. If you feel faint, you should pull to the side of the road if possible and do deep breathing exercises. Most panic attacks pass quickly, but the fear they leave behind may be the worst part.

Once a person knows his condition is panic disorder, he can stop believing that he's having a heart attack or going crazy. Knowing the problem is limited in time is usually helpful to the panic attack patient. Many of them can just wait for it to pass and then get back on the road. The main idea is not to become phobic of the road and driving.

I had one patient who always drove in the right lane on the highway so she could be ready to pull over if she had a panic attack. The possibility of a panic attack during driving caused her considerable worry. Once medication and psychotherapy worked on her, she became panic attack-free, but she still insisted on driving in the right lane and being worried. It took us many months concentrating on this issue before her habit could be changed.

Marvin's comments:

I had my first panic attack while driving, too. I had to fight not to become phobic of getting into my car and driving. The main idea is to obtain treatment as early as possible. Don't wait for the problem to cripple you.

Most panic attacks pass quickly, but the fear they leave behind may be the worst part.

57. The first time I had a panic attack, I was smoking marijuana. Now I don't smoke it anymore. Do you think my panic attacks could be relieved if I continue not to use it?

Different drugs may trigger panic disorder, or the disorder might start by itself without drug use. Marijuana is both an antagonist and agonist of serotonin receptors in different parts of the brain. Therefore, serotonin metabolism is affected, and panic disorder could start after a patient indulges in this drug.

Cocaine is a stimulant working on the epinephrine system. There are many case reports of people having their first attacks after cocaine smoking, snorting, or injecting. "Uppers" and other stimulants may have the same result as cocaine use. Even tobacco use or abstinence may trigger panic attacks. There is no guarantee that once a patient stops the drug use that he or she will return to normal and not have panic attacks.

One of my patients had her only panic attack the first time she tried marijuana. She didn't know what was happening to her at first, and thought that was what being "high" was like. She did not repeat the experience because it was so unpleasant. When she discussed it with friends, she learned that most people didn't have a panic attack when smoking marijuana. However, she never tried it again because it was so unpleasant, and she didn't know if it was a unique episode that would have occurred anyway, without the drug, or whether the marijuana triggered a panic attack.

58. The worst panic attack I ever had was while flying. Now I worry every time I step onto a plane. What can I do?

It is common to get panic attacks on airplanes. One patient told me how she ran off a plane one evening that she was sure was going to crash. Nothing happened to the plane. The patient realized afterwards that she was experiencing her first panic attack. Now, every time she boards a plane she takes 0.25 mg of Xanax®, which helps to keep her calm. If you have similar fears, you may ask your doctor to prescribe a small amount of a tranquilizer to help you through airplane flights. Alternatively, some people prefer techniques learned in cognitive behavioral therapy or **meditation**.

What you have experienced is called negative conditioning. Because you had a terrible panic attack during a flight, your mind had associated flying with the panic attack, even though the two events may not be related.

The Russian physiologist Dr. Ivan Pavlov studied positive and negative conditioning in the 1800s. Dr. Pavlov rang a bell and then gave meat to a dog. He did this several times until the dog associated his feeding with the ringing of the bell. Then he rang the bell without feeding the dog. The animal still salivated; although it received no meat, its mind had associated the two events. It would take several times of ringing the bell and not feeding the dog for the animal to stop associating the two events and stop salivating.

By taking Xanax® and avoiding a panic attack each time she boards the plane, the patient is breaking the connection between flying and panic attacks. Eventually, her association between the two events should fade out.

Meditation

Techniques using long, deep, slow breaths to calm the mind and help the body to relax; often used in conjunction with visualization techniques.

77

Cognitive behavioral therapy would teach the patient about the irrational views she might hold about flying inducing panic attacks. The cognitive behavioral therapist then would introduce more rational views about flying that the patient would then try to use when she boards a plane.

Using meditation you can do deep, slow breathing and visualize something positive in your history or imagination. This positive imagery can be anything: visualizing a sunset ocean scene and imagining yourself being there, watching the colors in the sky change, hearing the waves on the beach and the sea birds sing overhead, smelling the salty air. This visualization and working to slow and deepen the breathing increases your ability to relax. As your body relaxes, this decreases the anxiety that might trigger a panic attack.

59. My sister has schizophrenia and panic attacks. Is that possible?

Schizophrenia

Mental disorder due to organic changes in the brain that can cause delusions and hallucinations.

Delusions

Fixed, false beliefs.

Hallucinations

The apparent, often strong subjective perception of an object or event when no such stimulus or situation is present; may be visual, auditory, tactile, or involve smell or taste sensations.

Panic attacks may coexist with many other psychiatric diagnoses. Certainly schizophrenic patients may also have panic attacks. It is thought that 1% of the population of the world has **schizophrenia**. More and more we in the medical community understand that this disorder is due to organic changes in the brain.

People with schizophrenia usually have **delusions** (fixed, false beliefs) and/or **hallucinations** (the apparent, often strong subjective perception of an object or event when no such stimulus or situation is present; may be visual, auditory, tactile, or involve smell or taste sensations). Delusions may be paranoid ones, that is, the person has feelings of being harmed or pursued by characters in their delusions. The hallucinations tend to be auditory, meaning the patients will hear voices talking with them. These voices may seem to be originating from other people, the universe in general, or from inside the person's own head. The person with schizophrenia may also have a flat emotional state (termed affective flattening in the *DSM-IV*), disorganized behavior (childish or bizarre actions), and avolition (inability to initiate and pursue goal-oriented activities).

A schizophrenic person may still take the same medicines as any other person to stop panic attacks. These may be SSRI antidepressants or minor tranquilizers. There is a risk of triggering hallucinations or delusions if these patients take antidepressants, so sometimes it is better for them to take minor tranquilizers such as Klonopin® or Xanax®. Many patients with schizophrenia will already be on major tranquilizers, such as Zyprexa® or Risperdal®. Adding a minor tranquilizer may make a patient on major tranquilizers even more sleepy or tired, so it is preferable that they take an antidepressant instead.

60. My sister claimed that it was panic disorder that made her keep vomiting, but later we learned that she had bulimia. Can you explain this?

In **bulimia**, patients control their weight gain after binge eating by vomiting, or they may use laxatives, fasting, or excessive exercise. The vomiting is usually self-induced. Panic attack patients don't vomit very frequently, but they can feel nauseous or have abdominal pain. Excessive eating may occur in panic attack patients to calm themselves down. One patient of mine with panic disorder was actually phobic of vomiting. If she saw anyone doing this, it would induce a panic attack, so she tried her best to avoid anyone who was ill or vomiting.

Bulimia

A mental disorder in which patients control their weight gain after binge eating by vomiting, or they may use laxatives, fasting, or excessive exercise.

Your sister could very well have panic disorder and bulimia. Many psychiatric disorders tend to occur comorbidly (together).

Another patient of mine who had both panic disorder and bulimia did well by taking Zoloft®. In this way, she was able to eliminate both problems. Zoloft® (100 mg) left her panic attack-free, and over several months of medication and psychotherapy she was able to reduce her bulimic episodes from three times per day to one time per week. Eventually, over several years of treatment she stopped bulimia and only had a few panic attacks per year.

61. While taking Celexa® for my panic disorder, I found I had a decreased libido and decreased sensation during sex. What can I do about my decreased sexual appetite?

Unfortunately, all of the SSRIs, like Celexa®, are associated with sexual dysfunction. Other medicines, such as Wellbutrin®, can be added to treatment with Celexa® to counteract this side effect. However, sometimes the addition of something like Wellbutrin® can actually trigger panic attacks. Your psychopharmacologist has to work carefully with you to find a solution. Another answer is to lower the medicine to the smallest possible amount that won't allow panic attacks to break through, but that will allow normal sexual functioning. Still another plan is a "drug holiday," where one stops the medicine 24 hours before having sex and then immediately restarts the medicine after sex. Viagra® and similar medicines may also be used at the time of intercourse. Viagra® works by inhibiting an enzyme, thereby allowing more blood to reach the genital area. Both males and females may benefit from Viagra®. Yohimbine, derived from a South American plant, is sometimes as effective as Viagra®, but it has the disadvantage of inducing panic attacks for some people.

Marvin's comments:

I have a problem with sex on Celexa®. In fact, that's my only real side effect from the medicine. Not only did I have decreased sensation, I couldn't have an orgasm. I tried that drug holiday plan, but it didn't work because I had to stop my medicine for three days before my normal sexual functioning would return. By that time, Celexa® was completely out of my body and I would feel panicky, so I had to restart it. We tried adding other medicines but nothing really worked until I tried Viagra®. That worked, but I had to use 100 mg. I felt very embarrassed telling my date to wait twenty minutes before we had sex. If I were married it might have been different, but just dating made me feel I had to perform to the best of my ability. I discussed all this with my therapist, who helped me figure out that I was equating "being a man" with having an erection. Now that I'm more relaxed about it, I can usually use 50 mg of Viagra® with good results.

62. After I started having panic attacks, I found that I became very dependent on my mother. I feel ashamed of myself. How can I help myself to become more independent?

Many people start relying on others excessively once they have panic attacks. This may be O.K. at the beginning, but of course it can't last indefinitely. One of my patients asked her husband to travel everywhere with her when she started to have panic attacks. After awhile he found it stifling, plus he couldn't do his work. In therapy we analyzed dependency needs that she had. We discovered that she felt abandoned by her mother when she was a child and would cling to her in desperation when she was around. She had transferred this behavior to her husband when she became sick. Gradually, we weaned her away from being so dependent on her husband as her panic attacks decreased.

There are many psychoanalytical theories about dependency needs in panic attack patients. Many of them refer to the patient's belief that parents abandoned them in some way in childhood. One patient of mine remembers being lost in a big department store when she was four years old and shopping with her mother. It was a terrifying experience for her. Panic attacks started shortly afterwards. It was not clear if this was a real memory or a symbolic one that illustrated the way this patient felt about her mother.

She had a lot of shame about having panic attacks, too. Her understanding of panic attacks as a chemical imbalance helped her to relieve her embarrassment somewhat. This patient felt inadequate in many ways. Her single mother had made it clear to her that she was unwanted, saying to the patient, "If abortions were more available at that time, I would have had one." She often told my patient what a disruption of life the patient was for her. Perhaps the abandonment in the department store was unconsciously "intentional" on her mother's part. My patient felt ashamed and guilty that she was unwanted. We discussed these issues at length, and she was able to see that it wasn't her fault that her mother didn't want her. It wasn't her fault that she had a medical condition (panic disorder) either. These realizations helped her to feel less shame.

Talk with your therapist. She or he will be able to help you discover new insights about yourself. Once you can identify the personal history and/or reasons driving your fear, you can take steps to disengage that automatic response and develop new response behaviors that are more positive. In turn, you will find yourself operating in the world with more confidence and emotional tools to help you if you have another panic attack.

63. My panic attacks started after my father died. Is there any correlation?

Loss of any kind can trigger panic attacks because hormonal levels as well as **neurotransmitters** change with loss. Many patients can trace their panic attacks starting with the loss of a loved one. The best plan is to consult a psychiatrist at any signs of trouble after a significant death, like that of a parent, spouse, and child. Most people are aware that depression can be triggered by loss, but panic attacks being triggered by loss may be a new concept.

Psychotherapy allows you to access feelings about the loss of your father, and the medications will treat your panic attacks. Often people feel that they should get on with their lives and not dwell on losses. Recovery from your father's death will take at least six months. Hopefully, relief from your panic attacks will happen much sooner, since antidepressant treatment usually kicks in after four weeks.

If a loved one's death is impending, it's a good idea to start coping with it as soon as possible to avoid the shock aspect of the actual loss. This might consist of speaking about the loss with family, friends, and/or a therapist. Bereavement group therapy is usually beneficial. Often religious groups have helpful bereavement counseling.

Loss of any kind can trigger panic attacks.

Neurotransmitters

Upon stimulus, chemical agents are released in pre-synaptic nerve cells, and these agents travel through the synapse to the post-synaptic cells where they either stimulate or suppress them.

64. When I have PMS, I often get panic attacks. What can I do about this?

Some patients take SSRIs prophylactically to prevent panic attacks or depression during **premenstrual syndrome (PMS)**, which is basically a hormonal imbalance causing bloating, headaches, irritability, fatigue, and emotional instability. **Premenstrual dysphoric disorder (PDD)** is a more exaggerated form of PMS, and medication is strongly recommended for that condition.

Janet, a patient of mine, was on 20 mg of Celexa® every day for her panic disorder. A few days before her period, I instructed her to increase her Celexa® to 30 mg to combat her PMS. She did this for one year and found herself to be in a good mood on a daily basis as well as panic attack-free, even during her usual PMS times.

Another way to deal with PMS and panic attacks is to ask your gynecologist to prescribe birth control pills, if it's appropriate. Since the problem is caused by a hormonal imbalance, abnormal estrogen or progesterone levels, birth control pills may be able to restore that balance. Sometimes a well-balanced hormonal system can stop panic disorder, too.

Premenstrual syndrome (PMS)

A hormonal imbalance causing bloating, headaches, irritability, fatigue, and emotional liability.

Premenstrual dysphoric disorder (PDD)

A more exaggerated form of PMS, requiring medication.

65. When I was withdrawing from Klonopin®, I started having panic attacks. As a result I decided to stay on for another few months. How can I get off this drug?

All benzodiazepines should be withdrawn very slowly over a long period of time, especially in panic disorder patients. Some patients feel they can never get off a medication like Klonopin® because every time they try, they find they have panic attacks. Sometimes we can add an anticonvulsant or some other medication to help a person withdraw from Klonopin®. Often it is necessary to decrease the dosage slowly over many weeks. There is always a period of discomfort involved, and panic attacks are possible in the last few days of withdrawal.

I had a patient who was secretly taking twelve 1-mg Klonopin® pills per day in her attempt to control her panic attacks. She had been on the medicine for years and her system had grown resistant. Rather than share this information with me, she went from one doctor to the next getting prescriptions for Klonopin®. She was out of control. One day she couldn't get enough Klonopin® to keep up with her habit; she had a convulsion and was taken to the emergency room. I met her there, and she was forced to admit the extent of her Klonopin® habit. We hospitalized her and placed her on a slow detox schedule and Lexapro® (10 mg per day). It was very difficult for her to come off of the Klonopin, even in the hospital. After three weeks, she was stabilized enough to return home on the Lexapro® alone, which at that point still wasn't eliminating the panic attacks. Eventually (3 months later) the Lexapro® worked at 20 mg along with the addition of an anticonvulsant Topamax® (50 mg) to stop her panic attacks. Stories like this make doctors very cautious when prescribing Klonopin® for certain patients.

66. Is it better to take Xanax® or Klonopin® for panic disorder?

Taking any type of tranquilizer is difficult for panic disorder patients. These benzodiazepines should only be taken for limited amounts of time and used very sparingly. Klonopin® may be better because it lasts for

12 hours, that is, it has a longer half-life. Xanax® only lasts for three hours, so a patient needs a dose more quickly, which makes it more addictive. The best thing is to take these tranquilizers for short periods until an antidepressant can kick in (see Question 65).

Many times patients will prefer one medicine or another, because they feel better with it. If there are no contraindications (where the risk of taking the medication is inadvisable), doctors will prescribe that medicine. If a patient takes Klonopin®, it should be given only twice per day. A convenient schedule might be once at 8 AM and once at 8 PM for around-the-clock coverage.

67. I always thought that I had panic disorder because I was hiding my homosexuality. Could this have anything to do with it?

If hiding your homosexuality produced anxiety, then it could very well contribute to panic attacks. Anytime a person must hide something, he or she may feel worried and thereby activate certain chemical systems in the brain, such as the GABA and norepinephrine systems, which in turn can lead to panic attacks. Psychotherapy, either group or individual, will be of help to you.

One of my patients had his first panic attack when he went for an interview for a new job. He was 25 at the time, very presentable in a new, fashionable business suit and flowered tie. The employer was a prestigious, conservative businessman who was stern in his manner. My patient imagined that he was being scrutinized and silently criticized for his homosexuality. During the interview, he broke into a terrible sweat and his heart beat horribly fast. He felt as though he would die. Even though he had a panic attack for the first time, my patient said nothing and kept a poker face. He didn't think the potential employer knew what was going on. (He didn't get the job, and my patient found out later that this same businessman was gay, too.) But his anxiety triggered the attack, and my patient suffered from panic disorder from that point on. Those were the days when he didn't feel comfortable revealing his homosexuality. Nowadays he is "out" and not having panic attacks, either because his therapy and medications work or he is more comfortable with his identity.

68. Wherever I go into a social situation, I am afraid of having a panic attack. This makes me avoid many situations. Can you offer any help?

It is important to get therapy as soon as possible before you become phobic of social situations and acquire social phobia. Fear of panic attacks is one of the hallmarks of the disorder. Social phobia involves fear associated with all kinds of social situations, going outside of a familiar place, or many other innocuous conditions. Patients must resist avoiding these situations and endeavor to conquer their fears by going into them. Practicing social situations by your willingness to get involved with others, going outside for a walk, riding in an elevator, and facing other fears will help you learn that not all situations are scary, and enable you to build self-confidence.

Those with social phobia must make sure they don't have depression or a schizoid personality disorder. Going to a psychiatrist for treatment will help you figure out whether you have these conditions. If the patient has either of those two conditions, standard treatments for social phobia will not work. In the case of the patient with depression, it would help to take an antidepressant. The patient with schizoid personality disorder may not be able to conquer his or her fears of performance even after therapy.

One patient avoided going to parties or conferences where he would have to face many people. He was afraid that others would notice he was sweating or looking anxious. He had panic attacks in the past and was fearful that they would return. In therapy, we worked on his fears and discovered that he believed that other people were focusing excessively on him. His mother had done this when he was a child. I pointed out to him that he was an only child with whom his mother was overly concerned. Strangers and even colleagues were not that concerned with every nuance of his behavior the way his mother was. They were most interested in themselves and how they were doing. The patient could see the logic of this explanation, and he was able to apply it when he went out. It was a struggle for him to actually go out and attend events, but when he did, we both reinforced this behavior. I would reinforce it by crediting him every time he ventured out. He would reward himself by going to a movie or eating a favorite food, like popcorn. Eventually, going out became easier and easier until he looked forward to his outings.

69. I believe that it is a stigma to have panic attacks, so I don't want to tell friends or family. What should I do?

Many patients believe that panic attacks and, indeed, all mental illnesses are bad or shameful, and this is why they have trouble seeking treatment and getting help. Psychiatrists, psychologists, social workers, and other mental health professionals have been working for years trying to de-stigmatize mental disorders. Things are improving. Public figures such as movie stars, newscasters, and other famous people are stepping forward and discussing their depression and panic disorder. Millions of Americans take antidepressants and anxiolytics. People are out of the closet. Now the goal is to normalize it. Organizations such as NAMI and FAMI are endeavoring to de-stigmatize these mental disorders as well (see Question 100). If you could bring yourself to talk about it with others, you are helping people to understand and de-stigmatize panic attacks.

One patient thought long and hard about telling her boss that she had panic disorder. Finally, she decided that she would. When she did so, her boss was quite understanding and offered the patient time off if her panic attacks became severe. Another patient told her boss about her panic attacks and was met with a stony silence. A few months later when the chance to move into a supervisory position came up, my patient was overlooked for a colleague who was junior to her in years and service. My patient consulted an attorney and decided to sue her company. She is still involved in litigation, which is expensive, but the entire process has given her a sense of empowerment. The dilemma of telling your boss about your panic disorder can only be determined on a case-by-case examination of as many factors as possible.

Marvin's comments:

The stigma part bothers me, too. I don't go around telling everyone that I have panic disorder and I'm proud of it. Maybe if I had some physical disease like diabetes I'd be more up front about it. As it is, to admit to panic is to say you're a wimp or chicken about something. I want to be seen as a strong man so women will be attracted to me and men will feel I'm reliable. Who wants to be seen as weak and frightened? If I heard a male movie star whom I admire declare he has panic disorder, I wouldn't feel like joining him in his declaration. I would feel that with his money and position, he can afford to have it and say he has it. It would be like watching one of those male movie stars model jewelry—no one would think they aren't masculine—only that the rich and famous can get away with anything. If another guy admits he has panic disorder I might share that I have it too, but then again I might not, especially at work. The stigma is there, and it's not going away anytime soon.

70. Is there any exercise I can do to prevent panic attacks?

There is no specific exercise that will prevent a panic attack, but general exercise is a good idea. Those who never exercise may be more subject to surges of epinephrine, and their feedback systems will not work as well to offset chemical imbalances. Often, breathing exercises taught by psychologists, social workers, and yoga or tai chi instructors are helpful to some panic attack patients.

Breathing exercises consist of awareness of the rhythm and rate of breathing. Panic attack patients are notorious hyperventilators and shallow breathers. These patients can be taught to consciously breathe slowly and deeply. Yoga-like breathing may be useful. Simply concentrating on the breath, and slowing down its rhythm to deep, long, slow breaths will help you to relax your muscles and your mind. You should practice the new breathing as often as possible, because when a panic attack occurs, you will be ready to employ your breathing exercises without having to think about them. Instead, they'll be automatic.

One patient of mine claimed she could never breathe properly, so she couldn't learn any breathing exercises to help herself with her panic attacks. I sat her down and worked with her beliefs about her point of view. Eventually she saw that she had many preconceived notions about herself and breathing, and she was able to change. This woman often held her breath and then would breathe shallowly, which led to hyperventilation and panic attacks. If people allow themselves to vary their set patterns, they often experience relief of ingrained problems. It isn't easy to change behavior that has been in place for most of your life, but the proper attitude is to at least try.

71. Should I take a leave of absence from my highly stressful job?

I always encourage my patients to work if they can, because people with anxiety disorders need to have structure in their lives. Work is an easy way to provide daily structure. However, some workplaces are so stressful that they become debilitating. For example, stockbrokers, medical interns, and police officers often have such high stress that their bodies and minds are often on overdrive, with excess stimulation of the adrenergic system. In panic disorder patients, we are attempting to calm this system down, so in these cases work would be counterproductive.

People with anxiety disorders need to have structure in their lives.

I suggest taking a leave of absence for several weeks or trying to step down to a less stressful position. One example would be a police officer who gets a desk job for a while instead of being out in the field. For other, less stressful work, the panic disorder patient must train him/herself to take it much easier. They can attend group therapy for this purpose or work with an individual therapist who will guide them through relaxation techniques. Some individuals, especially high achievers and those with **obsessive-compulsive disorder**, find it more stressful not to work. If these types are at home they can become discouraged, melancholy, and even panicky. They should try to do their work or obtain some work, even if it's volunteer work.

Obsessive-compulsive disorder

Mental disorder that involves obsessions (thoughts, images, or impulses that occur over and over and feel out of control; the person finds them disturbing and intrusive, yet they don't make sense) and compulsions (certain acts are done over and over again according to "rules;" these rituals are performed to obtain relief from the discomfort caused by obsessions).

72. Ever since I've had panic attacks I've been hyperaware of my looks. It sounds odd, but I think my head looks too big and my body small and spindly. What is happening to me?

People do feel differently about their bodies and themselves after being diagnosed with various psychiatric disorders. If you really think you look weird, but everyone tells you that you look normal, you may have something called **body dysmorphic disorder (BDD)**. This is a preoccupation with imagined defects in appearance. Your concern has to be excessive, and it must cause you significant distress in social and work situations to make the diagnosis.

Body dysmorphic disorder (BDD)

A preoccupation with imagined defects in appearance; the concern must be excessive and cause distress in social situations.

I had one patient who thought he looked like a distorted dwarf. It was difficult to imagine what he was talking about, because to me (and most other people) he looked like a perfectly ordinary man. He was slightly below normal height, but otherwise not unusual. Yet every time he walked into a roomful of people he would get a panic attack, because he believed that people were staring at him and criticizing him. We worked very hard together two times per week in psychotherapy for many months to dissuade him from his false belief. He maintained his point of view even in the face of evidence proving that he was wrong. (I had him ask people how they felt about him, and they didn't report that they saw him as a dwarf.) The only thing that helped was Lexapro® (30 mg/day) after many weeks. This medicine decreased the panic attacks, but he still wasn't convinced that he looked quite normal.

Many patients have less drastic views of themselves. They may see themselves as too fat or with a big nose. In reality, they have none of those features, but they are exaggerating their perceived defect in their minds. Through therapy, many patients acquire realistic views of themselves through testing of their images with others or looking at themselves more objectively. They are often surprised to learn that they look quite normal and that their points of view in terms of physical appearance are distorted.

73. Should I tell my other doctors that I have panic disorder? I think that they'll treat me differently and tell me that all my ailments are in my head.

It is important to tell other physicians that you have panic disorder, especially if you're taking medicines. Many medicines don't go together well, so if your cardiologist, for example, wants to give you a medicine that makes your heart race, he should know you suffer from panic disorder, so he won't give you that medicine that would make your heart race and make you think you're having a panic attack. There are usually alternatives. Many people hide panic disorder from their other medical doctors because they don't want them to think every sickness is stemming from mental disorders. Unfortunately, even some doctors may believe that is true. This is the stigma that was discussed in Question 69. Many times I will call other physicians and explain about a patient's panic attacks. Most doctors are glad to be updated about this disorder. They may have studied it 30 years ago when they attended medical school, but have been so busy keeping up with news in their own specialty that they don't have time to review the latest information about psychiatric problems. If medical doctors aren't up to the latest information, you can imagine how the lay public may have misconceptions about panic. However, I do believe it is a panic attack patient's obligation to inform other doctors, and staff in hospitals, emergency rooms, and clinics of his or her condition as well as any medicines taken.

Marvin's comments:

I told my general practitioner about my panic disorder. His response showed me that he didn't know anything about it. He sat me down and tried to talk to me about panicky feelings. I said "Don't worry, doc, I have a therapist who goes though all of these things with me." He said, "What are you so anxious about?" I explained that I was anxious about a lot of things—that it was just my nature. Panic attacks were different than my normal anxiety. I told him about the faulty alarm system in the brain. I think he can use a copy of this book. It's surprising that regular doctors don't learn more about psychiatry. I'm sure half of the patients they're treating have more psychological than physical problems. Anyway, I will continue to tell my other doctors about panic disorder even if they don't completely understand me.

74. How do I tell my children about my panic attacks? Shouldn't I tell them?

If children are very young, that is, under five years, they won't be able to understand that their mother or father is incapacitated in any way. At that age they see parents as god-like and all-knowing. Any defects in the caregivers are frightening to them. If they witness you struggling with a panic attack, try to do deep breathing or relaxation exercises, and assure them and yourself that everything is O.K. Of course everything is O.K. What is the worst that can happen from a panic attack? Fear and running from a situation. If children are older than five years, panic disorder can be explained to them in a very simplistic way. You can say, "Mother is not feeling well now. Her heart is beating fast and she's dizzy, but she'll be fine in a few minutes." It is better to speak about it than to not speak about it. If anything is hidden, its significance multiplies many times, particularly with children. They can sense something is happening. You can explain that it's a chemical imbalance that causes an episode of fear. If you have trouble revealing your panic attacks to your older children, you can ask your psychiatrist to see you and your children in a session and impart the information then. Sometimes family therapy is an appropriate way to give information. Then your spouse and other family members are invited in to a session. Many patients have found these family sessions very helpful.

75. My psychiatrist had to switch me from one medicine to another and then another. The one I'm on now (Lexapro® 20 mg/day) took a long time to kick in, and I only have about 80% relief from my panic disorder. What should I do?

Sometimes one medicine won't work, so a psychiatrist must discontinue that one and try another and still another. The process can be very frustrating for patients because they just want to get better and return their lives to normalcy. My advice is to remain as patient as possible. Medicines, especially antidepressants like SSRIs, have to be tried for at least five weeks at certain dosages. Shorter time periods and lesser dosages often don't work, and they are considered inadequate trials. If you go to another doctor he or she will just have to try that medicine again, so try to stick it out the first time. There's no way that your psychiatrist can tell which medicines will work for you except for trial and error and past clinical history. Sometimes what worked at one time won't work the second time.

If you find a medicine that works well, try to stick with it.

The nervous system is a constantly adaptable and changing system that we in the medical community don't fully understand. It's not unusual to have several attempts at treatment with different medicines and combinations of medicines. If you find one that works well, try to stick with it. If a medicine works 80%, that is excellent. Many times medicines will only work 20% to 30% of the time. Any relief is welcomed, but of course you can keep trying different ones until you find a satisfactory solution.

76. I'm afraid of needing to be hospitalized in a psychiatric unit for panic attacks. Can that happen?

It is very rare for patients to be hospitalized for panic disorder. Most cases are handled on an outpatient basis. If someone is hospitalized, it is usually for some other psychiatric condition that occurs with panic disorder. This could be major depression, bipolar disorder, a schizophrenic break, or another problem. Panic attacks could be the predominant symptoms, but they probably won't be the cause of admission to a psychiatric hospital. The amount of fear that you have about this possibility is the same as the usual worries experienced by other panic attack patients. They are always worried that something terrible will happen to them as result of their panic attacks.

I had a bipolar patient who became manic and needed to be hospitalized (see Question 28). One night she waited outside her dormitory and propositioned random men to have sex with her. Her usual good judgment was certainly impaired. My patient tended to be on the prudish side, staying with one boyfriend since her senior year of high school. Her manic behavior was quite unusual and dangerous for her, so I decided to hospitalize her. At first she protested, claiming that I was taking away her sexual freedom. In the hospital she also complained of panic attacks. Of course, that was not her primary problem, and if panic attacks had been her only complaint, I would not have hospitalized her. When she came down from her manic high, she thanked me for hospitalizing her and sparing her further shame from her irrational behavior.

Marvin's comments:

I was afraid I'd be taken to a mental ward too when my panic attacks first started. You really believe that you've flipped out. You try to grasp the idea that you are having such tremendous panic, and the most obvious explanation seems to be that you've gone crazy. Fortunately, it's not true. You haven't turned into a raving lunatic who can never control himself again. You are just having discrete episodes of anxiety. They will stop by themselves in a short while and then you'll take a medicine that will banish them further. Since I've started having panic attacks, I've met two other people who have them. Neither one was hospitalized. One person only gets them once or twice a year, so she doesn't even have to take medicine. The other person took Prozac® and that worked for him.

77. After 9/11, I wandered away from home and was unable to remember who I was or where I belonged. It was a horrible experience. My panic attacks began at that time, too. Can you explain?

Dissociative fugue

A mental disturbance in which a person travels away from home and can't recall his or her past and is confused about identity; often occurs in wars and traumatic events.

You had an episode of what is called **dissociative fugue**. This is a disturbance in which a person travels away from home, can't recall his or her past, and is confused about identity. It is a rare condition and can occur during wars or great catastrophes like 9/11. People wish to withdraw from horrible experiences and painful emotions.

A history of head trauma, alcohol, or other substance abuse may predispose one towards this disorder. Temporal lobe epilepsy may also result in dissociative fugue.

Usually this fugue state only lasts hours to days, but after a severe trauma like 9/11, panic attacks can be triggered, too, which then can last for years. It sounds like your experience of the September 11th event triggered both conditions. You should seek psychiatric treatment, which can consist of hypnosis, medications, and psychotherapy.

I had a patient who forgot who she was and where she belonged after her mother died. Her mind was trying to deny the reality of her mother's death. She also experienced her first panic attacks at this time. Her family found her and brought her back home. It took her several weeks to return to her normal state of mind and remember everything. The problem was that her panic attacks continued and had to be treated with several medications before they resolved.

78. I've been told that I have multiple personality disorder with four different personalities. One of these personalities has panic attacks and the others don't. Why is this true?

Multiple personality disorder is now termed **dissociative identity disorder (DID)**. This condition is usually triggered by childhood trauma, like physical and/or sexual abuse. What happens is that various aspects of an individual cannot cohere into a single integrated person, because of the severe disturbances the patient experienced in the past. Parts of the person are broken into different personalities or identities, each one with its own unique way of perceiving the environment and the self. These different identities will take control of a patient at different times. People cannot recall various events when they are in the different personalities, so they will

Dissociative identity disorder (DID)

A mental disorder that is usually triggered by childhood trauma, like physical and/or sexual abuse; the severe disturbances the patient experienced in the past create different identities that control the patient at different times. Formerly called multiple personality disorder.

experience time distortion, headaches, hearing voices, being told by others about strange behavior, or finding other clothes or items from the other personalities. Some patients even have different prescriptions for eyeglasses and different clothing for different personalities. Often a person will have panic attacks in one identity but not in another, because one personality can experience certain emotions or aspects of things and another cannot. The best plan would be to engage in psychotherapy and pharmacotherapy to relieve the panic attacks. Any background severe enough to cause DID can definitely trigger panic attacks.

Marvin's comments:

Sometimes I feel that I have different personalities, but Dr. Berman assures me that I don't have DID. I guess if you could believe that the part of you having a panic attack is a different personality than the "real" you, that might help you separate yourself from the problem. However, I believe we're supposed to integrate the different aspects of ourselves into a whole person. Therapy allows us to get in touch with our various feelings and our different attitudes. In that way we have more access to ourselves. Maybe I was separated from my feelings in the first place and that's how I started having panic attacks.

79. I have asthma. Many times when I am having an asthma attack I feel a panic attack coming on, too. What can I do?

Asthma

An inflammatory disease of the lungs characterized by reversible (in most cases) airway obstruction.

Asthma can often trigger panicky feelings. In addition, some of the stimulant medications used to treat asthma can cause panic attacks. The first step is to inform the treating asthma doctor, usually an internist or pulmonologist, that you have panic disorder as well.

Once that doctor knows, then he or she can prescribe more steroids and fewer stimulants. Also, you should learn breathing exercises to regulate your breathing and attempt to control both conditions. Allergy season may be a particular problem, and anti-allergy medications without stimulants should be employed.

A patient of mine had her first panic attack during a bout of asthma. After she had calmed down from the asthma attack, she felt her heart racing and had a feeling of impending doom. This happened to her several times before she consulted me. I prescribed 10 mg of Celexa® once per day. This medication went nicely with her asthma medications and she soon felt quite well, although she did worry about having panic attacks for a long time afterwards.

80. I am always assessing myself to see if I'm O.K., to check if I am about to have a panic attack. Is there anything I can do?

A constant state of vigilance is not the best thing for a person recuperating from panic disorder. People have probably told you to relax for a long time. Of course you can't just relax. Your nervous system doesn't allow it. You must learn to relax and not obsess about your condition, because paradoxically such anxiety can trigger attacks. Cognitive behavioral therapy, meditation, hypnosis, psychotherapy, medications, and biofeedback can all be useful to you in your endeavor to relax.

I hypnotized a patient and gave her a pleasant beach scene to keep in mind when she felt anxious. She could picture the bright blue skies with white seagulls flying overhead. I had her imagine walking through warm, soft sand with her bare feet. Salty sea breezes ruffled her hair. Whenever she felt overwhelmed by office stress, I told her to close the door of her office, sit back with closed eyes and see herself on this sunny beach. It worked. She found that she was able to abort some panic attacks with this technique.

Marvin's comments:

I was always checking myself to see if I'm O.K. The slightest unusual pounding of my heart would make me believe I was having a panic attack again. Through therapy I learned to be less neurotic—to leave myself alone. I think it started with my mother always worrying about me. I was sick a lot as a child, so she stayed home from work and took care of me. We bonded through my sickness. In therapy I learned to stop monitoring my every breath and heartbeat. All my physical tests were normal. If something was wrong I would let my doctors find it. My job was to leave myself alone, do therapy, and take my medicine.

81. Why do I fear dying when I have a panic attack?

Fear of dying is a very common fear that many anxious people have even when they are not having a panic attack (see Question 7). Anxious patients fear the unknown, and what could be more unknown than death? As people die, they might have a flood of adrenaline similar to panic attack patients. The good news is that I've never heard of a person dying from a panic attack.

Anxiolytics

A type of medication that combats anxiety.

It's important to control fear with cognitive behavioral therapy techniques, mental imagery, and positive thinking (see Question 41). Medications, especially **anxiolytics**, are helpful to reduce this fear.

Most of us are in a state of denial about death, so if people focus on death it is considered unusual. Panic attack patients are focused on death when they worry about it. Psychoanalytically it may be related to abandonment anxiety. For young children, abandonment is almost the equivalent of death, since they are helpless and can't take care of themselves. Panic attack patients may be fixated on these early fears, which may be reawakened during panic disorder. This is the reason that psychotherapy is helpful, since it allows patients to deal with these unconscious issues and bring them to consciousness. Then a new strategy can be developed and implemented to alleviate the anxiety.

82. I took yohimbine for my sexual dysfunction and had a panic attack. Should I be concerned about this?

Yohimbine, which is derived from a South American plant, promotes norepinephrine release, thereby helping with sexual dysfunction. However, panic attack patients who already have malfunctioning of their norephinephrine-epinephrine neurons via the locus ceruleus cannot tolerate an added stressor, so they may obtain panic attacks from yohimbine. Perhaps it would be better if you stayed away from this drug and tried Viagra® or one of the other medications that promote more blood into the genital area. Viagra® and other similar medicines would not induce panic attacks. Yohimbine is known to sometimes trigger insomnia or manic episodes.

Yohimbine

An alkaloid medicine derived from the South American plant, *Corynanthe yohimbi*, that blocks β-adrenergic receptors; has alleged aphrodiasic properties.

83. When my father had panic attacks they gave him propanolol, which helped. When I tried that drug, it didn't help. What's going on?

Propanolol

A β-adrenergic blocker once used as a medication for panic attacks before newer and better medications.

Propanolol is a β-adrenergic blocker. It was used before we knew that panic attacks could be controlled with anti-depressants. If we return to the theory of noradrenergic overload (see Question 6) and a false alarm system going off, then it is understandable why blockage of this system would control panic attacks. However, it is not so simple. Some people have other systems, like the serotonin or GABA systems, that are out of order. Propanolol over the long run (months) can cause depression. Since we have much better medicines now, I suggest that you try one of the SSRIs.

However, propanolol is useful in controlling social phobia (see Question 68). One patient of mine was a violinist with panic disorder and social phobia. When he stepped onto the stage his hands would tremble with fear of his performance, and he worried that he would have a panic attack. Propanolol (10 mg) given twenty minutes before the concert helped him to control his fears and to stop the actual trembling that he experienced in earlier episodes. When he told other members of his orchestra what medicine he was taking, he was shocked to learn that 70% of his colleagues used the same medicine to control their shaking, too.

84. I once had a panic attack that lasted all day. Is that possible?

It's possible but unusual to experience a panic attack for an entire day, because most panic attacks last 5 to

30 minutes. Remember: For a panic attack to be a panic attack, it has to have 4 out of 13 symptoms listed in Table 1 (see Question 1). I've heard other patients complain that their panic attacks lasted all day. Sometimes generalized anxiety can last all day or for several days (see Question 3).

Another patient told me that she had a panic attack that lasted several days, but when I questioned her very carefully, I discovered that her symptoms did not constitute true panic attacks. Instead, she had generalized anxiety for those days. Knowing that it was not constant panic attacks helped to keep her calm. Panic attack patients can exaggerate sometimes, much to their own detriment. If a person views a glass of water as being half empty, that pessimism can work against him or her. It is much healthier to cultivate a positive view of the glass as being half full.

85. I tried many other medicines, but now my psychiatrist has put me on an MAOI called Nardil®. It works, but I'm frightened that I'll get a hypertensive crisis reaction. What can I do?

Monoamine oxidase inhibitors (MAOIs) are one of the standard treatments for panic disorder. MAOIs, like Nardil®, have been around for many years. They work by stopping the breakdown of monoamines (like serotonin and norepinephrine) by irreversibly inhibiting the enzyme monoamine oxidase. There are newer MAOIs called **reversible inhibitors of monoamine oxidase** or RIMAs that allow the enzyme to be reversibly inhibited; that is, if the enzyme needs to be used, then the MAOI will bounce off and allow the breakdown of

Monoamine oxidase inhibitors (MAOIs)

A standard medication for panic attacks. They work by stopping the breakdown of monoamines (like serotonin and norepinephrine) by irreversibly inhibiting the enzyme monoamine oxidase.

Reversible inhibitor of monoamine oxidase (RIMA)

A medication for panic attacks that allows the enzyme monomine oxidase to be reversibly inhibited.

monoamines. This is important because when the MAOI cannot reverse itself, large amounts of dangerous mono-amines like tyramine can build up and cause a hypertensive crisis, which in the worst case scenario could mean a stroke. People on MAOIs must eat a diet restricted from high tyramine-containing foods, such as cheese or red wine. If they eat cheese, they risk a stroke because eating cheese increases not only wanted monoamines, like serotonin and norepinephrine, but also unwanted ones like tyramine, too. It is difficult for patients to stick to this diet, so MAOIs are usually used after all other treatments fail. If your psychiatrist has already given you TCAs, SSRIs, and so on, and these medications failed, you might be left with MAOIs. If that's all that works, you have to try them.

To avoid a hypertensive crisis reaction, always ask what foods contain when dining out. Sometimes waiters will not tell the truth (or know the truth). One patient of mine on an MAOI ate in a Chinese restaurant and asked the waiter if the chicken chow mein contained any monosodium glutamate (MSG). He was assured by the owner of the restaurant that there was no MSG used in the restaurant, but after he ate his dinner he got a terrible headache. When he went to the emergency room (ER), his blood pressure measured at a dangerous level of 200/170. This was the beginning of a hypertensive crisis. Fortunately, he was in the ER and the doctors were able to lower his blood pressure, so he didn't have a stroke, which is the concern during these crises when the BP rises so high because the patient cannot metabolize tyramine.

86. What are the differences between medicines like Tofranil® and Prozac®? I took Tofranil® for a long time and felt much more stable, but I was always constipated so my doctor put me on Prozac®.

Tofranil® is a tricyclic antidepressant (TCA; refer to Table 2 in Question 38). These medicines are known as the classic antidepressants. They are imipramine (Tofranil®), amitriptyline (Elavil®), doxepin (Sinequan®), desipramine, nortriptyline, etc. All of these medications contain at least a three-ring nucleus chemically. Some of them even contain four rings (three and a side chain), such as, amoxapine (Asendin®). These medicines have been in use for over 30 years and are quite reliable for treatment of panic disorder as well as major depression, GAD, OCD, and other mental disorders. They work by reducing the re-uptake of norepinephrine and serotonin, thus providing more of the monoamines needed to combat panic and other disorders. They also block acetylcholine and histamine receptors, which produce adverse effects such as dry mouth, constipation, blurry vision, and weight gain. The newer selective serotonin reuptake inhibitors (SSRIs)—fluoxetine (Prozac®), sertraline (Zoloft®), and paroxetine (Paxil®)—have been available since 1988. They are as effective as the TCAs and are easier to use because they have fewer side effects, like constipation. The SSRIs inhibit serotonin reuptake and basically don't affect the other monoamines such as norepinephrine and dopamine. They also don't have anticholinergic, antihistaminergic, and anti-adrenergic side effects. However, they can cause weight gain and sexual dysfunction. Both TCAs and SSRIs are useful medicines for panic disorder. Many doctors have switched their patients from TCAs to SSRIs. However, sometimes patients have found that the older medicines were more stabilizing and were able to eliminate panic attacks better than the newer SSRIs. If this is true for you, be sure to tell your doctor.

87. I had a terrible time going off Paxil® after I was on this antidepressant for one year. In fact, I had thought my panic attacks were gone, but they came back with a vengeance as I was withdrawing from Paxil®. Now I'm afraid to even try to go off. Can anything be done?

Working with a good psychopharmacologist may help. Paxil® is one of the most difficult antidepressants to stop. Many patients are discouraged when they try to withdraw from it. I usually decrease the medication in my patients very slowly over a long period of time. For example, if you were on 30 mg of Paxil®, I would ask you to take 25 mg for one week, then 20 mg for one week, 15 mg the week after, and so on. As you can see, you would only be decreasing by 5 mg per week. This usually works for most people, although it's too fast for some. Each patient must work closely and tailor treatment with his or her psychopharmacologist. We in the medical community don't think that antidepressants cause withdrawal symptoms per se, but many people are extremely uncomfortable going off of some medications, and they can have a reoccurrence of panic attacks. Patients can experience dizziness, nausea, headaches, and/or stomachaches while decreasing Paxil®.

One patient of mine claimed he was having withdrawal from Paxil® for seven months after he stopped it. I had no choice but to believe him. I added a small amount of Prozac® (5 mg) to help him with symptoms of dizziness, malaise, and insomnia. This worked well, and then I withdrew him slowly from Prozac®.

88. Is there an increased risk for Alzheimer's if you have panic disorder?

To date there has been no association between having panic disorder and developing **Alzheimer's disease**. There are panic disorder patients who have Alzheimer's and Alzheimer's patients with panic attacks. The two conditions are not mutually exclusive. Alzheimer's disease is a degenerative disease of the brain that is associated with neurofibrillary tangles and plaques, which decrease cognition and cause premature senility and mental deterioration.

An elderly patient of mine was diagnosed with Alzheimer's and placed into a nursing home when she became too easily disoriented and would wander away from her apartment. In the nursing home, it was discovered that she was having a reoccurrence of her panic disorder, which had been resolved in the past. We re-added Lexapro® 5 mg to her other medications and she improved. In a patient like this, psychotherapy often is not productive because the patient's memory is so impaired that she can't use cognition to help herself. Benzodiazepines, like Klonopin® or Xanax® would also be inappropriate, because they would make the patient too drowsy and might decrease her capacity to think.

Alzheimer's disease

A degenerative disease of the brain that is associated with neurofibrillary tangles and plaques, which decrease cognition and cause premature senility and mental deterioration.

109

89. When my allergies kick up, I always take antihistamines. Will these interfere with Zoloft®?

You may take Zoloft® and various antihistamines on the same day. As with most medications, it is a good idea to take two medicines at different times of day or night. For example, if you are taking Claritin® as well as Zoloft®, you may take your Zoloft® after breakfast and then take your Claritin® after lunch. In this way, the two medicines can be absorbed separately and they will not interfere with each other. Pharmacodynamics, that is, how different chemicals interact, can be complicated, so if you have any doubts, be sure to ask your psychopharmacologist.

One allergy patient complained that her Zoloft® was not working to counteract her panic attacks, which had been the case before allergy season. I instructed her to take the allergy pill in the morning and Zoloft® at night. This worked well, and she was soon relieved of both her allergies and her panic attacks.

Marvin's comments:

One antihistamine to be careful of is Benadryl®. When I tried that, it gave me a panic attack. I tried Claritin® while taking Celexa® and that didn't have a bad effect on me. As Dr. Berman says, the best thing is to take any two medicines separately. Take Celexa® in the morning and then take Claritin® at night. I don't have allergies often, but when they do strike me, I can be pretty miserable. I guess this is another reason why you should tell all your doctors about panic disorders and the medicines you're taking. They need to adjust their medicines with respect to the ones your psychopharmacologist is giving you.

90. Why are so many antidepressants and other medicines associated with liver problems? My doctor told me I have a liver problem, so he was reluctant to prescribe Prozac® to me.

All medicines are filtered through the liver and/or the kidneys. If you have a problem with your liver, like **cirrhosis** or **hepatomegaly** (enlargement of the liver), then you may have trouble filtering and metabolizing medicines. You may have to take 50 mg of Zoloft®, for example, rather than 100 mg like most people. If you were to attempt to take 100 mg you might feel nauseated, have diarrhea, and other adverse effects. Your doctor needs to monitor you carefully and get liver function tests. You may still use medicines like Prozac® or other SSRIs, but in much smaller doses.

Some people have such damaged livers that they cannot take medications without becoming toxic. These patients may need liver transplants. A few medications are filtered through the kidneys, which need to be in good condition for a patient to be able to tolerate those medications.

Cirrhosis

End-stage liver disease, resulting in jaundice, hypertension, fibrosis, and enlargement of the liver; can be due to chronic alcoholism or congestive heart failure, among other disorders.

Hepatomegaly

Enlargement of the liver.

91. Is there any truth to everyone worrying about increased suicidal risk with antidepressant use?

Any patients who have depression, panic disorder, or other mental disorders are at a greater risk than the general population for suicide. When people are ill and without medication they sometimes don't even have the strength to try to commit suicide. However, when they first receive medication in weeks one through five, before the antidepressant can actually kick in, they might have enough agitation and energy to hurt themselves. We in the mental health community have known for a long time that this is true. These are dangerous weeks of treatment. Most mental health professionals are aware, and they are particularly vigilant about the suicidal risk then. Lately, the media has discovered these facts, and many alarmists have risen up protesting against antidepressants. Unfortunately, this frightens patients away from taking medicines. As if the stigma and anxieties surrounding panic disorder weren't enough, we also have to worry about misinformation! Now patients have to worry about the "black box" warnings about suicidal risks with antidepressant use. If you feel suicidal, you should immediately inform your therapist, psychiatrist, other physicians, trusted family members, or friends. There are suicide hotlines as well. If all else fails, you may call 911 and ask for an ambulance to take you to an emergency room. Once there you'll be able to speak with an on-call physician, probably a psychiatrist, who will be able to help you resist your suicidal wishes either by immediate counseling or hospitalization. We know how difficult it is to reveal such feelings to others. However, it is essential that you do so, rather than act out on impulses.

92. What can I do about the fifteen pounds I've gained from taking my antidepressants?

Unfortunately, we have discovered that one side effect from practically all antidepressants is weight gain over time (months to years). I have advised my patients to watch for weight gain and attempt to keep the pounds off the best they can through exercise and diet. Many medication changes may be made if you are aware of weight gain.

First, dosages can be lowered to the minimum amount that will still eliminate panic attacks. Then other medicines, like Wellbutrin®, may be added to offset weight gain. The mood stabilizer and anticonvulsant, Topamax®, may be taken with an SSRI like Prozac® or Zoloft®.

A patient complained that she had gained twenty extra pounds after six months of treatment with Zoloft®. I reduced her dose from 200 mg to 150 mg without causing her to have a reoccurrence of panic attacks. However, she still found it impossible to lose the weight, so I added 50 mg of Topamax®. Once she had that medication and did some intense dieting, she was able to shed the extra pounds.

Marvin's comments:

I've also gained about ten pounds from my medication. I've stopped eating desserts and I try to cut down on the carbs. Exercise is what keeps me on track. After a basketball game or a good workout, I feel great. I'm going to try to do more of that and less of just sitting indoors watching TV.

93. Does it make sense to have a social worker psychotherapist and a psychiatrist to take care of my medications?

Many times patients work in a team approach, with a social worker, psychologist, or psychotherapist for behavioral therapy in conjunction with a psychiatrist or psychopharmacologist for medication. The combination can be a good one as long as the two professionals have a system of communication with each other. If they don't, one can counteract the other.

For example, I saw a patient whose therapist was a social worker who constantly insisted that the patient ask me for more and more of the Prozac® I had prescribed for her. It wasn't appropriate, so I called the social worker and explained that more Prozac® might tip the balance and cause our patient to get more panic attacks. The social worker hadn't understood that information, and she thanked me for educating her. After that we worked smoothly together. The patient benefited because she wasn't confused about our opposing opinions.

It is much more difficult for a psychiatrist to work with a lay therapist, that is, someone who doesn't have a LCSW, CSW, or PhD training and degree. Lay therapists may be appropriate for some patients, but they have limited educations and do not understand about medication and conventional psychotherapy. If they do the wrong thing in treating a patient, they probably can't be held liable for their mistakes the way professionals can; health care professionals can be sued and/or their licenses to practice can be revoked.

94. Do I need to get a CT scan or an MRI to really have a diagnosis of panic attacks made?

At this point in our technology, obtaining a computerized tomography (CT) or magnetic resonance imaging (MRI) scan won't help in the diagnosis of panic disorder. Of course, they can help the doctor to rule out brain tumors and cerebrovascular disorders.

95. When I was on HRT alone (no other medications), I felt fine, but as soon as I stopped it, my panic attacks came back. I can't take HRT anymore because of the new studies and my strong family history of breast cancer. What can I do?

Many women have decided to stop **hormone replacement therapy (HRT)** since the 2002 studies were published because of the negative study results and side effects of women who took the hormones to relieve the symptoms of menopause. As a consequence, we in the healthcare community have seen many women, who had only used HRT and were in remission from mental disorders, have a return of panic attacks, major depression, GAD, and so forth. Estrogen and progesterone, the two main female hormones that are given in various combinations in HRT, usually have a positive effect on the central nervous system (CNS). This is not always true, otherwise we would not have so many more women than men affected by panic disorder and depression.

However, when estrogen and progesterone are withdrawn, either naturally in menopause or artificially in hysterectomies and oophorectomies, a return of symptoms of panic or depression can recur. Antidepressants are usually the best solutions to panic disorder and/or depression if a woman cannot tolerate HRT. I suggest that women should consult with a psychopharmacologist and start an SSRI like Lexapro®. Most women have no problems with these medicines. Sometimes the most difficult symptom to control is insomnia after women stop HRT. Therefore, a very sedating antidepressant may have to be used, such as Paxil®.

Hormone replacement therapy (HRT)

Estrogen and progesterone, the two main female hormones, are given in various combinations in different HRTs to relieve the symptoms of menopause.

96. Now that I'm finally panic attack-free, how can I live an enjoyable life and not worry about the attacks returning?

The most difficult thing to do after the panic attacks have stopped is to learn to enjoy life again. Most patients always maintain some degree of vigilance and fear that their panic attacks will return, even when they are panic attack-free.

Psychotherapy, of course, is the most popular way to get back on track. You must analyze what is disturbing you in the first place and cope with it. Most panic attack patients are notorious suppressors of their feelings. In therapy, people learn to get in touch with all of their feelings, including sadness, anxiety, depression, happiness, shame, and rage. A lot of people do not feel comfortable expressing any of these emotions. Our society does not promote people emoting all over the place. How would we conduct business or take care of our families, if we burst into tears or into raucous laughter at the slightest provocation? Thus, as a group, we are encouraged to hold everything in and perhaps deal with it later. Often that later never comes, and we never give ourselves time to grieve over our father's death or celebrate our birthdays.

By designating a therapy time, we at least give ourselves permission during that time to deal with our feelings. Other ways to learn to enjoy ourselves would be to get back into participating in sports that we enjoy. Basketball, baseball, swimming, walking, and tennis are excellent ways to relax ourselves and gain back a sense of pleasure. Other people may try yoga, meditation, or tai chi. Creative endeavors like writing, painting, and music should be encouraged as well. Identify the things you enjoy doing and do them.

97. How do I find a good psychiatrist to treat my panic attacks?

If you live in a big city, you can call the psychiatry department of the best hospitals and ask them to recommend a psychiatrist specializing in anxiety disorders. Another way would be to ask friends and family members to recommend a psychiatrist who can make the diagnosis and then recommend another person for psychotherapy or medication if that particular doctor is not a therapist or is exclusively a psychopharmacologist. Sometimes attending lectures on panic disorder might connect you to experts. In New York City there is MDSG (Mood Disorders Support Group), which conducts seminars, lectures, group therapies, and recommends doctors. You may have similar societies in your town. The Appendix lists more resources and suggestions.

98. How do I find a psychotherapist for me?

Remember, there are many professionals who can provide psychotherapy for you. These include social workers, nurses, psychologists, psychiatrists, some priests and rabbis, and occasionally qualified lay therapists. Once you have verified a person's credentials, consider where they have studied psychotherapy and for how many years, what kind of degree they have, and determine their philosophies and types of psychotherapy they offer. Then, for the most important aspect that many people skip, you must determine if their personalities suit you. In a way, it's almost like being on a date. It's important to try different therapists to see which one suits you. If you find the person so obnoxious that you can't stand to hear his voice, then don't choose that therapist. There is no reason

It's important to try different therapists to see which one suits you.

to suffer with someone whom you believe is irritating. Psychotherapy should be enjoyable to a large extent.

99. What about alternate therapies like hypnosis?

Hypnosis

An artificially induced trance-like state in which the subject is highly susceptible to suggestion, oblivious to all else, and responds readily to the commands of the hypnotist.

Hypnosis is an artificially induced trancelike state in which the subject is highly susceptible to suggestion, oblivious to all else, and responds readily to the commands of the hypnotist. There are some patients who may benefit from hypnosis, but not very many. Most psychiatrists believe that panic attacks stem from a chemical imbalance and disturbed transmission of neurons in the brain. Hypnosis is not traditionally thought of as a way to alter brain chemistry or transmission. It may be helpful for cessation of smoking, weight control, dealing with conversion disorders, and recovery of certain memories.

Patients should be warned about various nontraditional therapies that they read about on the Internet or hear advertised on TV. Many of these are just "get rich" schemes on the part of charlatans.

A patient of mine went off his medications and changed his entire lifestyle after he became involved with an organization that he found on the Internet. His family despaired because they saw him falling back into depression and panic disorder without his medicine or therapy. He could not withdraw from the group and their activities because they were able to draw him in, as do many cults. He became suicidal, and I had to hospitalize him (not just for panic attacks). In the hospital, we were able to de-condition him, and he finally consented to go back on his medications to good effect. This particular story ends well, but many do not. It is always a good idea to thoroughly check out an organization or particular therapy that is offered on the Internet before getting involved. Most certainly, do not stop taking your medication(s) without the supervision of your doctor.

100. Where can I get more information?

There are many organizations and web sites that offer information about panic disorder. A few helpful resources are listed in the Appendix that follows.

Do not stop taking your medication(s) without the supervision of your doctor.

SURVIVING

Appendix

Organizations

American Psychological Association
750 First St., N.E.
Washington, DC 20002-4242
www.apa.org

American Psychiatric Association
1000 Wilson Blvd. #1825
Arlington, VA 22209-3901
www.psych.org

Anxiety Disorders Association of America
8730 Georgia Ave., #600
Silver Spring, MD 20910
www.adaa.org

Association for Advancement of Behavior Therapy
305 7th Ave., 16th Fl.
New York, NY 10001
www.aabt.org

Freedom From Fear
308 Seaview Ave.
Staten Island, NY 10305
www.freedomfromfear.org

Get Mental Help, Inc.
19206 65th Place, N.E.
Kenmore, WA 98028
www.getmentalhelp.com

National Alliance for the Mentally Ill
Colonial Place Three
2107 Wilson Blvd., #300
Arlington, VA 22201-3042
www.nami.org

Web Sites

www.anxietypanic.com
www.nimh.nih.gov
www.factsforhealth.org
www.expert-help.com
www.panicattacks.com

Telephone Number

Panic disorder information and free brochures:
1-800-64-PANIC

Glossary

A

Adrenaline: A hormone secreted into the body that stimulates physiology that deals with fear and anxiety. Also called epinephrine.

Adrenergic: Having to do with nerve pathways in which transmission is with epinephrine (adrenaline) or norepinephrine.

Affect: Feeling tone; if sustained it becomes mood.

Agoraphobia: Anxiety about going or being outside and/or avoidance of certain places or situations where it might be difficult or embarrassing to escape.

Alzheimer's disease: A degenerative disease of the brain that is associated with neurofibrillary tangles and plaques, which decrease cognition and cause premature senility and mental deterioration.

Antidepressants: The best medicines to stop depression and panic attacks; non-addictive and may benefit the nervous system in many ways.

Anxiety attack: An episode of fear that is not as defined as a panic attack and doesn't have to occur out of the blue as most panic attacks do.

Anxiolytics: A type of medication that combats anxiety.

Asthma: An inflammatory disease of the lungs characterized by reversible (in most cases) airway obstruction.

B

Behavioral therapy: A type of treatment aimed at changing overt behavior by a variety of techniques such as systematic desensitization, relaxation training, flooding, participant modeling, and positive and negative reinforcement.

Benzodiazepines: A type of drug used for short-term treatment of panic attacks to decrease anxiety; potentially addictive.

Bipolar disorder: A mood disorder where the person experiences both an elated state (hypomania or mania) and at other times depression.

Blush: A sudden and brief redness of the face and neck due to emotion.

Body dysmorphic disorder (BDD): A preoccupation with imagined defects in appearance; the concern must be excessive and cause distress in social situations.

Bradycardia: A slow heartbeat, under 60 beats/minute.

Bulimia: A mental disorder in which patients control their weight gain after binge eating by vomiting, or they may use laxatives, fasting, or excessive exercise.

C

Caffeine: A powerful central nervous system stimulant found in coffee, tea, and cola; should be used with caution in panic attack patients.

Cirrhosis: End-stage liver disease, resulting in jaundice, hypertension, fibrosis, and enlargement of the liver; can be due to chronic alcoholism or congestive heart failure, among other disorders.

Cocaine: An addictive central nervous system stimulant that potentiates catecholamines and causes euphoria; panic attack patients should avoid this substance.

Comorbid: When two disorders exist at the same time.

Conditioning: The process of acquiring, developing, educating, establishing, learning, or training new responses in an individual.

D

De-condition: To change or eliminate a conditioned (learned) response.

Delusions: Fixed, false beliefs.

Depersonalization: Not feeling like oneself, feeling dissociated from the self and the body; often occurs in panic attacks.

Depression: A state of a lowered mood, usually with disturbances of sleep, appetite, suicidal thoughts, etc.

Derealization: Feeling of unreality or that one's surroundings are unreal; often occurs during a panic attack.

Diagnostic and Statistical Manual of Mental Disorders, Fourth Edition (DSM-IV): Reference textbook of classifications used by mental health professionals to diagnose people with mental disorders.

Dissociation: Thoughts and feelings are not accessible to conscious awareness; a "spaced-out" feeling.

Dissociative fugue: A mental disturbance in which a person travels away from home and can't recall his or her past and is confused about identity; often occurs in wars and traumatic events such as the 9/11 act of terrorism; usually is temporary.

Dissociative Identity Disorder (DID): A mental disorder that is usually triggered by childhood trauma, like physical and/or sexual abuse; the severe disturbances the patient experienced in the past create different identities that control the patient at different times. Formerly called multiple personality disorder.

E

Echocardiogram: An ultrasound record of the heart.

Electrocardiogram (EKG): An electrical record of the heart, which shows the heart's integrated action currents; useful test to rule out cardiovascular problems or disease.

Ephedra: An amphetamine-like drug which can cause anxiety and should be avoided by panic attack patients.

Epinephrine: A chemical hormone released in the body after a stress stimulus (also called adrenaline) it is a "fight or flight" chemical that makes a person able to flee or fight an enemy or danger.

F

Flooding technique: One type of behavioral therapeutic technique in which a patient is exposed to his worst fear all at once in an effort to lessen or eliminate the fear; not recommended for panic attack patients.

G

GABA system: The system of neurotransmitters in various parts of the brain that are responsible for inhibiting neurons. If the GABA system is not working well, nerve cells are not turned off (inhibited) when they should be, and excess stimulation can occur that results in panic attacks and other unwanted events. (See also **Gamma aminobutyric acid**, below.)

Gamma Aminobutyric Acid (GABA): The most abundant central nervous system amino acid that works to inhibit neuronal transmission; it may malfunction in panic disorder.

Gene: A DNA sequence that codes for a protein, genes are the biological basis of heredity.

Generalized Anxiety Disorder (GAD): A constant, excessive worry with restlessness, fatigue, irritability, and sleep disturbances; GAD patients can also experience their minds going blank, muscle tension, and feeling on edge.

H

Hallucinations: The apparent, often strong subjective perception of an object or event when no such stimulus or situation is present; may be visual, auditory, tactile, or involve smell or taste sensations.

Hepatomegaly: Enlargement of the liver.

Hippocampus: A region of the temporal lobe of the brain that controls learning and memory.

Hormone replacement therapy (HRT): Estrogen and progesterone, the two main female hormones, are given in various combinations in different HRTs to relieve the symptoms of menopause or hysterectomy.

Hyperthyroidism: Increased thyroid hormone secretion causing anxiety, weight loss, etc.; sometimes it can mimic panic attacks.

Hyper- or hypoglycemia: Too much or too little, respectively, sugar in the blood.

Hyperventilation: Excess respiration that can occur during a panic attack and may bring about a dizzy or faint state.

Hypnosis: An artificially induced trancelike state in which the subject is highly susceptible to suggestion, oblivious to all else, and responds readily to the commands of the hypnotist.

Hypochondriasis: A condition in which one believes and worries that one is ill when one is not.

Hypothalamus: An area of the brain below the thalamus involved in the control of the nervous system and certain hormones.

L

Limbic system: Brain structures, including the hypothalamus, responsible for smell, emotions, and behavior.

Locus ceruleus: Collection of blue-appearing neurons in the pons containing a large number of noradrenergic nerve cells; the area of the brain that might be falsely triggered during panic attacks.

M

Meditation: Techniques using long, deep, slow breaths to calm the mind and help the body to relax; often used in conjunction with visualization techniques.

Mitral valve prolapse (MVP): Excessive backwards movement of the mitral valve leaflets into the left atrium of the heart during ventricular systole, sometimes giving mitral regurgitation; MVP has been associated with panic attacks.

Monoamine oxidase inhibitors (MAOIs): A standard medication for panic attacks. They work by stopping the breakdown of monoamines (like serotonin and norepinephrine) by irreversibly inhibiting the enzyme monoamine oxidase.

N

Negative conditioning: See **Conditioning**.

Neuron: A nerve cell, the basic cell unit of the brain and spinal cord.

Neuroreceptors: A structural protein molecule on the nerve cell that binds to a specific factor, such as a neurotransmitter.

Neurotransmitters: Upon stimulus, chemical agents are released in the presynaptic nerve cells, and these agents travel through the synapse to the post-synaptic cells where they either stimulate or suppress them.

Nocebo reaction: When a patient feels frightened of a medicine and so has a bad reaction to an innocuous substance.

Nonsteroidal anti-inflammatory drugs (NSAIDs): A large number of drugs exerting an active effect to reduce or eliminate inflammation (sometimes analgesic and antipyretic actions, as well); examples include aspirin, ibuprofen, indomethacine, and naproxen.

Noradrenaline (or norepinephrine): A catecholamine hormone secreted from the adrenal gland, similar to adrenaline but having different effects on bronchial smooth muscle and cardiac output.

Norepinephrine: A catecholamine hormone stored in the adrenal medulla that is secreted in response to hypotension and physical stress; used pharmacologically as a vasopressor.

O

Obsessive-compulsive disorder: Mental disorder that involves obsessions (thoughts, images, or impulses that occur over and over and feel out of control; the person finds them disturbing and intrusive, and yet they don't make sense) and compulsions (certain acts are done over and over again according to "rules;" these rituals are performed to obtain relief from the discomfort caused by obsessions).

P

p450: An enzyme system in the liver, which helps to break down various medicines and foods during metabolism.

Palpitations: A sensation of the heart pounding or pulsing, often experienced in panic attacks.

Panic attack: A discrete episode of anxiety, defined extensively in Table 1 in Question 1.

Pheochromocytoma: A very rare condition where the hypertensive patient has a benign tumor of the medulla of the adrenal gland; the patient produces a lot of adrenaline or epinephrine, which raises the blood pressure and causes palpitations and sweating, symptoms that make a person believe he or she is having panic attacks.

Phobia: An objectively unfounded, morbid dread or fear that arouses a state of panic; used in combination with the object that inspires the fear.

Placebo reaction: Where a person has a positive effect from an innocuous substance such as a sugar pill.

Posttraumatic stress disorder (PTSD): After being exposed to a traumatic event (like 9/11, Oklahoma City bombing, war, rape, etc.), experiencing feelings of being threatened by death or serious injury to the physical integrity of self or others. The emotional response must involve intense fear, helplessness, or horror. Afterwards, the traumatic event is persistently re-experienced by distressing recollections, dreams, flashbacks, and psychological distress to internal and/or external cues that represent the traumatic event. Also, PTSD patient must have a physiological reactivity when re-exposed to things surrounding the event (such as sweating or rapid heart rate).

Premenstrual dysphoric disorder (PDD): A more exaggerated form of PMS, requiring medication.

Premenstrual syndrome (PMS): A hormonal imbalance causing bloating, headaches, irritability, fatigue, and emotional liability in women.

Propanolol: A β-adrenergic blocker once used as a medication for panic attacks before newer and better medications.

Prophylactic: Prevention of a disease or process that can lead to a disease.

Psychiatrist: A medical doctor (MD) specializing in psychiatry, the treatment of mental diseases and disorders.

Psychologist: A PhD professional who can provide behavioral and other types of therapy, administers and analyzes

psychological tests, but cannot prescribe medication (see psychiatrist).

Psychopharmacologist: Psychiatrist who specializes in prescribing medicines for mental disorders.

R

Receptor: A protein molecule on the surface of a cell that receives and binds neurotransmitters, hormones, etc.

Reversible inhibitor of monoamine oxidase (RIMA): A medication for panic attacks that allows the enzyme monomine oxidase to be reversibly inhibited; that is, if the enzyme needs to be used, then the MAOI will bounce off and allow the breakdown of monoamines, such as tyramine.

S

Schizophrenia: A psychiatric disorder characterized by psychosis with delusions and hallucinations.

Selective serotonin reuptake inhibitor (SSRI): A type of antidepressant that doesn't allow serotonin to be taken up again by neuroreceptors, thereby causing more serotonin to be present to the neurons, which decreases panic attacks; includes drugs such as Prozac®, Zoloft®, Paxil®, Celexa®, Luvox®, and Lexapro®.

Serotonin: A neurotransmitter that may be decreased in depression and panic attacks.

Sleep terror disorder: Characterized by abruptly waking from sleep with a panicky scream, feelings of intense fear—a rapid heartbeat, shallow rapid breathing, and sweating—the person is unresponsive to others trying to comfort him or her and usually has amnesia for the episode. The symptoms of fear, a rapid heartbeat, deep breathing, and sweating are similar to those with a panic attack, but the unresponsiveness to comfort and amnesia are unique to sleep terror disorder.

Social phobia: A marked and persistent fear of one or more social or performance situations, exposure to unfamiliar people or to possible scrutiny by others. The fear is that the person will act in an anxious way that will be embarrassing or humiliating.

Social worker: A licensed clinical social worker (LCSW) or certified (CSW) graduate health care professional who can provide behavioral and other types of psychotherapy, but cannot prescribe medication (see psychiatrist, psychologist). Treatment focus can be on the whole individual as well as family and/or groups.

Syncope: Fainting, loss of consciousness.

T

Tachycardia: A fast heartbeat.

Temporal lobe epilepsy: Epilepsy in which epileptic foci are located in the temporal lobe of the brain.

Thalamus: A part of the brain that has to do with pain and some emotions.

Tricyclic antidepressants (TCAs): Includes Tofranil® and Elavil®. Among the first types of medication used to treat depression, popular before SSRIs came into wide use; can be used to treat panic disorder.

V

Vasodilation: A widening of the blood vessels, at the skin surface, causing a flushed or blush; may be due to an increase in adrenaline.

Vasovagal response: Relating to the action of the vagus nerve on the blood vessels, can lead to fainting.

Vigilance: A constant stressful state that strains the nervous system, leading to anxiety, panic, and other disorders.

Y

Yohimbine: An alkaloid medicine derived from the South American plant, *Corynanthe yohimbi*, that blocks β-adrenergic receptors; has alleged aphrodiasic properties.

Index

Italicized page locators indicate a figure;
tables are noted with a *t*.